A BEGINNERS GUIDE TO GOING

Cover design by Rachel Joy Olsen.
Back cover photography by K.J. Pictures, 4-13
Studios

All inquiries may be addressed to:

Living Meatless Nutrition & Wellness/R.J.O. Wellness
& Associates.
Calgary, Alberta

E-mail: livingmeatless@gmail.com
Website: www.livingmeatless.com,
www.RJOWellness.com

2019.

Disclaimer

This book is only meant to be a guide. The information is not intended as a substitute for consultation, evaluation or treatment by a medical professional, registered dietician or nutritionist.

The services, and information, provided by Rachel Joy Olsen, or Living Meatless Nutrition & Wellness, are not intended to be, and should not be, construed as a substitute for medical advice nor can they be represented as a guarantee of improvement of specific conditions or weight loss.

All meal plans, recipes and supporting information and guidance are developed solely for your personal use and may not be reproduced for publication or for the personal or commercial use of others without permission.

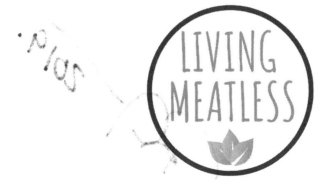

Table Of Contents

Going Meatless

If you are already living a meatless or vegan lifestyle you will find this book to be a refresher. However; if you are eating a traditional North American diet and are curious about how a meatless diet may help support your nutrition and health goals, this book will serve as an inspiring introduction to the lifestyle and its benefits.

Imagine if this one change is what catapults you into a completely new and upgraded life.

I used to eat meat. I understand that letting go of the foods you love can be very challenging and, at times, even heart-breaking. However, this decision is far more significant than just giving up your favourite foods. It is one that will not only positively impact your life but the lives of many others and the planet.

I commend you for being here. It takes great courage to changes, especially when it means going against some social norms. However; going meatless has never been easier. People all over North America are starting realize the benefits of this lifestyle and the endless options of delicious food.

Although many people think that making this transition is hard, it's easier than you think when you're prepared, have all the information you need to do it correctly and are ready for it.

If I can do it, so can you.

I know how hard, and even scary, it can be switch to a meatless lifestyle. That's why I'm committed to providing you with as much information as I can in this book, and online at **www.livingmeatless.com.**

You will notice I often use the term meatless, rather than vegan. The word vegan often comes with a negative connotation and to some being vegan feels limited and restrictive. However, after you read this book I hope you feel confident in embracing a meatless lifestyle in whatever way is best for you.

When people who eat meat find out I am vegan they sometimes assume that I'll judge them for their lifestyle choices. They think I will give them a lecture on how being vegan is the only way to live.

When I first became vegan, I was a little preachy at times but I soon figured out this was no way to inspire people to make changes in their lives. The best way is to live my life, be a role model and inspire others by being true to myself.

For me, being vegan not only means embracing a healthy and compassionate lifestyle, it represents something bigger. It is my mission to reduce preventable chronic disease and human suffering, save animals from a life of torture and prevent further destruction of the planet. Being vegan is the best way I know how to contribute to making a positive impact.

I am often asked, "what's the difference between a vegetarian, plant-based and vegan diet?"

It's simple.

A vegetarian diet is one where a person chooses to to no longer consume the flesh of animals but still eats animal products like milk and eggs.

A plant-based diet is one where a person eats only plant foods but may still use products that have been tested on or made from animals.

A person who identifies as a vegan not only eats a diet of only plant-based foods but also eliminates the use of products tested on or made from animals such as leather, fur and feathers.

Unfortunately, the word vegan has also been negatively twisted as a result of extreme animal activism, and in some cases, extreme judgement and hate crimes against non-vegans. That is why when I first became vegan, even just saying the word would cause people to roll their eyes and get defensive. This is why I now choose the term meatless, or plant-based. However, I no longer want the word vegan to have a negative connotation so I came up with an

7

acronym using the letters to represent something more positive.

Visionaries
Ever
Growing in
Abundance and
Nourishment

To me, this definition represents a group of individuals who love and respect themselves and who have compassion and empathy for other humans, animals and the planet. These people see a prosperous future for the human race, and the planet, and are willing to do what it takes to preserve it.

I believe this definition is one you can use as a daily mantra to keep you focused on why you have decided to go meatless.

The knowledge you gain from this book will allow you to achieve your best health and greatest potential, have more compassion and make a positive contribution to the planet.

This book is for you if:

- you are curious about how to go meatless but not sure how to do it in a healthy way;

- you think going meatless is intimidating and restrictive;

- you are tired of having low energy, dealing with health issues, or excess weight, and are ready to experience a level of health you never thought possible;

- you want to learn how to make meatless recipes that will taste as delicious as your traditional favourites;

- you want to know how to develop a healthy meatless meal plan;

- you love animals and no longer want to contribute to their suffering and exploitation; and

- you care about our beautiful Mother Earth and no longer want to contribute to her further destruction.

What can you expect from this book?

Although, you may think it will be hard to shift to a meatless lifestyle it isn't as difficult as you think. However, if you try to change everything all at once, it will be overwhelming. If you take it one step at a time it will be easier and enjoyable.

This book will help simplify this lifestyle. Once you learn about the new and delicious foods you get to eat and the results you will achieve you will wonder why you didn't make the switch sooner.

You may choose to use this book a few different ways:

- as a kick-starter guide to help you embrace a vegan lifestyle;

- read it all the way from cover to cover and let the ideas take their time to sink in;

- read it one chapter at a time and implement the ideas as they are presented to you; or,

- keep the book handy and refer to it as often as you need to remind you of the reasons why this decision is important to you.

Chapter 1:
Your Story

Before you get started on this journey, take a moment to reflect on your life. Write your story.

To help you get started with this process, consider these questions:

1) How has your health been in the past?

2) How is your health right now?

3) Do you love animals?

4) Do your actions support your love for animals?

5) Do you care for this planet?

6) Do your actions support your care for this planet?

When you dig deep, look back at your past behaviours and examine your current ones, it may be a little disheartening.

When I first became vegan and considered my choices I had at the time, I was sad and disappointed. My actions didn't always reflect what I thought were strong values. However, when I made the decision to change it became easier. Once my actions fully represented my values and beliefs it all came together.

Start developing your story now because once you make the switch to a meatless lifestyle you will have an inspiring story to tell others. Perhaps your story, from where you were to where you are now, will help someone else make this change.

My heart opens a little more when people tell me I inspired them to go meatless. It means they have made the brave decision to take care of themselves, no longer exploit animals or contribute to the destruction of this planet.

My Story

For many years I struggled with digestive distress and food and sugar addictions. It wasn't until I discovered the healing power of plant-based nutrition that things started to change.

My transition was a slow one. I was vegetarian for about 10 years before I fully converted to a vegan diet. I did as much research as possible and took it one-step-at-a-time. I will never forget the day I finally made the decision to stop eating red meat.

It was my mother's birthday. I had just filled my face full of beef ribs. As I sat back, stuffed to the brim, my stomach began to scream in pain. It was so uncomfortable I actually thought something was seriously wrong with my intestines. It felt like they were all twisted up.

A few weeks before this gluttonous meal, I had learned about an interesting book called, *Eat Right For Your Blood Type* by Dr. D'Adamo (D'Adamo 1996).

In his book, Dr. D'Adamo's theory is that food, beverages and activities affect people with certain blood types differently. He suggests that if you follow his guidelines, based on his research, it will be easier to manage your weight, reduce your risk of disease and have more energy.

According to Dr. Adamo's theory, my blood type A, fared better on a mostly plant-based diet. Considering how my stomach ached after eating all those ribs I began to think there was something to this theory.

The problem was that a plant-based diet was not something my family had ever spoken about. I had no idea what to do except for the suggestions in the book. Luckily, my mom and grandmothers always had a garden, so I was blessed to know and love fresh vegetables. But there was always meat, butter, milk and cheese on the table.

After reading more of Dr. D'Adamo's book I was starting to seriously consider modifying my diet. However, at that point I didn't feel I had enough information about how to eat a plant-based diet so my body would stay healthy and strong.

I had been told my entire life that meat, cheese, butter and milk were good for me and needed to be part of my diet. Learning this new way of living meant contradicting everything I had ever been taught by my family and health professionals.

I started slowly on my journey to a vegan lifestyle by taking Dr. D'Adamo's advice. The first thing I did was stop eating beef and pork.

Not eating pork was easy for me as I'd never really enjoyed pork. Even though I grew up with the smell of bacon and eggs frying on the stovetop on Saturday mornings, I figured I could live without it if it meant feeling better.

Beef was a little harder since I enjoyed eating a perfectly cooked filet mignon fresh off the barbecue in the summer. However, I had a reason to avoid meat so I was determined to remain committed.

After a few weeks, I noticed that my stomach didn't feel as bloated so I decided to take the next step and stopped eating poultry. Even though I enjoyed eating turkey for Thanksgiving and Christmas dinner, I wanted to see what would happen if I completely cut it out of my diet.

14

By refraining from eating beef, pork and poultry my digestion started to improve. However, I was still experiencing stomach pains and couldn't figure out why.

Then, I went for lunch with a good friend. He noticed that after I ate salad I complained of a stomach ache. I thought that was silly since vegetables shouldn't cause me any digestive distress. He pointed out that every time I eat salad there's cheese on it. Maybe the problem was dairy.

I was horrified that he might be right. I loved dairy. I could live on only cheese, yogurt and cheesecake. What if it were dairy? Would I be able to give that up to feel better?

My friend challenged me to cut out dairy for one week just to see what would happen. I accepted his challenge. Mostly to prove him wrong.

What I discovered was my stomach pains were virtually non-existent within just one week of cutting out dairy-based foods. I could no longer deny the fact that dairy was likely the biggest culprit for my digestive distress.

During this little experiment, I began to research more about dairy and how it is made. I couldn't believe what I discovered.

The industry itself seemed to exploit animals more than any other. After all, to get cows' milk the female cow must be pregnant and her baby prevented from drinking her milk. I also learned that the hormones and antibiotics given to the cow, during and after her pregnancy, as well as any infections she suffered were passed to her milk. It's no wonder humans who consume dairy have adverse side effects.

I made the decision to eliminate dairy and learned how to replace my dairy favourites with non-dairy options. It wasn't as hard as I thought. I grew quite fond of plant-based milk and yogurt and learned how to make raw vegan cheesecake and other favourite desserts using non-dairy ingredients.

Before embarking on this journey to plant-based eating I had been training for figure competitions, which are a division of women's female fitness and bodybuilding. The problem was I couldn't tolerate the meat-heavy diet. Now that I had switched to a plant-based diet I wanted to see if there was any way I could train for competition eating nothing but plant-based foods.

I spent some time searching for plant-based coaches online. Although, years ago, they were not that easy to find, I soon found a coach who was a raw-vegan fitness athlete and model.

I had no idea what a raw-vegan diet was but learned that it's someone who eats a fully plant-based diet and does not cook any food at temperatures greater than 118 degrees Fahrenheit.

I connected with him and he agreed to help me on one condition. I had to follow a fully raw-vegan diet. I knew I had a lot to learn about this diet but I was up for the challenge.

He asked me to take things to the next level, which meant cutting out fish and eggs, the only animal products I was still eating.

Cutting out fish and eggs was a little harder for me as I loved a nicely cooked salmon and going for brunch to enjoy a cheese and pineapple omelette. However, since letting go of cheese, omelettes weren't as good anymore and I figured I could refrain from eating fish at least until the competition was over.

My new coach sent me a raw-vegan meal plan and asked me to follow it as closely as possible. I have to admit, it was pretty easy since the majority of the foods I was required to eat were fruits and vegetables with some nuts and seeds. But I craved warm food, especially since it was winter in Canada.

For the most part, I was committed to the diet when I was at home. However; when I went out for dinner I would sometimes sneak a bite of fish.

I did my best and learned as much I could from my coach about the health benefits of being entirely raw-vegan. Over the next few weeks, I started to feel better. My skin cleared up, I had more energy and I was leaning out quicker than ever before.

As I continued to learn about the benefits of being vegan, including not supporting the cruelty of animals, staying vegan was easier.

Because I was feeling healthier and more vibrant I wanted to advance my knowledge and share this lifestyle with others so I became a certified raw vegan nutritionist and chef.

I made delicious food from recipes I found in vegan cookbooks and discovered new ingredients like nutritional yeast, which tastes like cheese.

I had so much fun developing my own recipes and sharing these dishes with my friends and family. People started asking me for the recipes and encouraged me to write a cookbook.

So I did.

The Magic of Living Nutrition was my first self-published cookbook that sparked my love for sharing new recipes. This book helped many of my friends and colleagues try new plant-based foods and transition to a vegan lifestyle. I still get compliments on the recipes in that book.

Over the years, people have asked me if being vegan is hard. At the beginning it was more difficult because I was not confident in my reasons for wanting to become vegan. So, I would sneak a piece of fish or eat eggs here and there and then feel badly about it.

However, the more I learned about the animal industry and the torture that millions of animals endure so humans can use their bodies for food, clothing and other products, remaining vegan became easy.

I also learned that the agricultural industry is responsible for much of the destruction of the environment. For me, this is unacceptable and difficult to support.

Am I perfect? Not at all. But I do my best and I always remember my reasons for making the switch. Now, after many years of being vegan I couldn't imagine my life any other way.

When people ask, and they have, "are you still doing the vegan thing?" I laugh because they don't get it. Being vegan is not only the way in which I eat. It's who I am.

That is why it is my mission to help people make the transition to a healthy, whole-food and plant-based lifestyle.

It is wonderful to see many other people who are also passionate about this lifestyle offering recipes, education and support to those who are vegan or want to become vegan.

More and more vegan restaurants are opening up and many mainstream restaurants offer plant-based menus, making it easier for vegans to enjoy dining out with friends.

Becoming vegan is one of the biggest movements in the world right now.

I encourage you to embark on this exciting and life-changing journey. Being vegan will not only fuel your body for better performance and health but also allow you to make conscious and compassionate choices that will have a positive impact on the world.

Chapter 2:
Know Your Why

An abundance of research has been done to prove that eating a whole-food, plant-based diet will result in better health. Even the American Dietetic Association released this position statement in a July 2009 publication:

> *"It is the position of the American Dietetic Association that appropriately planned vegetarian diets, including total vegetarian or vegan diets, are healthful, nutritionally adequate, and may provide health benefits in the prevention and treatment of certain diseases. Well-planned vegetarian diets are appropriate for individuals during all stages of the life cycle, including pregnancy, lactation, infancy, childhood, adolescence and athletes (Craig, Mangels, ADA 2009)."*

When people embrace a diet rich in plants the results often include weight loss, more energy, prevention and better management of disease.

21

Experts continuously prove that a plant-based diet is the healthiest way to eat and is the best strategy, along with regular exercise, to prevent disease.

Some of my favourite plant-based experts to learn from include:

- T. Colin Campbell, researcher and author of The China Study

- Dr. B. Clement, director of Hippocrates Health Institute

- Dr. Gabriel Cousins, physician, author and founder of the Tree of Life Centre,

- Dr. C. Esselstyne, physician and author

- Dr. M. Greger, Physician, author and speaker

After making the switch to a plant-based diet many years ago I have seen health benefits, such as weight loss, more energy and clear skin. I've never looked or felt better in my life and my mission is to share this longevity secret and to inspire others to embrace this lifestyle.

The reasons people choose a whole-food, plant-based diet differ for everyone. However, truly knowing your why is the secret to making this a successful lifestyle choice.

The top reasons people choose to make the switch include:

1) The Animals

Although health was my reason for making the switch it's not the main reason why many people are compelled to transition to a vegan lifestyle.

Studies show the number one reason people make the switch to a vegan lifestyle is because of their love of animals.

People who have become and remained vegan for this reason, have compassion in their hearts for all animals and don't want to contribute to the suffering and slaughter of any sentient being.

To most people, meat is nothing more than a product that is purchased in a grocery store or at a butcher. The reality is that meat, dairy and eggs come from living beings that have been raised specifically for slaughter or to harvest their products.

"But they're happy animals that live on beautiful green farms," you may say. The sad part is this is far from the truth. Most animals are raised for food. The demand for meat, and other animal products, is astronomical and unsustainable for local farms to supply. Enter the factory farm.

A factory farm is a large operation that houses thousands of animals, including cows, chickens and

23

pigs. To maximize production, prevent and treat diseases and to enhance growth and food output, these animals are often pumped full of antibiotics and hormones. These products are then transferred to the bodies of the people who consume the flesh of these animals and has been shown to result in various health problems.

Statistics show that billions of animals are killed each year worldwide for food (Sanders 2018). This does not include wild game hunting. Many of the animals killed are subjected to unnatural conditions, like small crates, are force-fed food like the flesh of other animals (fed to vegetarian animals) and genetically modified food that these animals cannot digest. This makes them sick and as a result they endure extreme pain and suffering.

Many animals are dragged screaming to their deaths. Sometimes limbs are broken, flesh is torn and other painful and stressful situations arise when these animals are sentenced to death. Often the killing process fails, forcing these animals to be stabbed, or shot in the head with a bolt gun more than once and in many cases are cut open or skinned while still alive.

Not only are the living situations for these soulful beings inhumane, it's unhealthy for us to consume and unethical for us to support. This is a topic of debate, that for me, seems like a no-brainer. Animals are living, breathing beings and deserve more from us.

Think about this for a moment. Do you have an animal? A pet you think of as part of the family? Now picture your sweet little pet going through a factory farm as I have mentioned above. Doesn't it concern you?

In most countries, if any form of animal abuse happens to household pets people are outraged, yet everyday millions of other intelligent, sentient beings, such as cows, pigs and chickens, are tortured in the most unforgivable ways.

Remember, if you purchase factory-farmed products these animals will continue to live, and die, in this nightmare.

> **"He who is cruel to animals becomes hard also in his dealings with men. We can judge the heart of a man by his treatment of animals."**
> **~ Immanuel Kant ~**

PETA (People for the Ethical Treatment of Animals) is an animal rights organization that works hard to educate people about the mistreatment of animals. Although some people consider PETA to be a radical organization, based on some of their tactics to create awareness about animal abuse, they are a strong voice for the animals. For this, I am thankful they exist.

Some people say animals are not intelligent so it's okay to eat them. In one of PETA's handbooks, "PETA Vegan Starter Kit," the organization talks about how intelligent many animals, such as pigs, fish, cows and birds, really are (PETA, 2019).

How Intelligent Are Animals?

Pigs: According to the information provided by PETA (2019), pigs have been shown to have personalities much like dogs and have been shown to be smarter than our canine friends. They can learn to sit, jump, fetch and respond to many other commands.

On factory farms, sows (female pigs) are confined to small crates to give birth. After giving birth, they feed their babies for a short time before the piglets are tragically taken away to live their own life of solitude and torture until they are slaughtered.

Pigs raised for meat are slaughtered in the most inhumane ways. If you treated your household pet this way you would be criminally charged.

Cows: Research has shown that cows can learn to do various tasks including open gates, operate a drinking fountain and show excitement upon accomplishing a task. They are very loveable creatures. Yet these beautiful animals, if raised for meat, are confined to filthy feedlots that disrupt their natural social structure leaving them unhappy and unhealthy.

Dairy cows have their babies ripped away from them within hours of birth so that humans can drink the milk. They are artificially inseminated to keep their milk flowing, hooked up to painful metal machines and forced to stand for hours to give milk.

Baby calves are torn away from their mothers and sent to live in small dark pens for a few weeks before being slaughtered and their meat sold as veal.

A cow can live upwards of 30 years, yet the average dairy cow lives to be only about four years old. When these cows are no longer able to produce milk, they are discarded in often painful ways left to suffer until they die (PETA, 2019)

Fish: Studies show that fish are fast learners and form complex relationships with one another. Many fish are able to count, tell time, garden and use tools to assist them in finding and eating food.

The idea that lobster and crab cannot feel pain is a myth. They can feel pain and have been shown to take action to avoid repeating a painful experience. Despite these facts, lobster and crab are routinely ripped apart, cut and boiled alive. Fish are suffocated or killed by decompression when exposed to pressure changes as a result of being rapidly pulled out of the water.

The fishing industry also kills millions of birds, turtles, marine mammals and plant life each year due to the use of fishing nets (PETA, 2019).

Birds: Newborn chicks have been shown to count to five by the time they are only two weeks old, use mathematical calculations to navigate using the sun and understand that objects hidden from view still exist. These are all concepts that human babies don't even grasp until they are at least one.

Turkeys have problem-solving reason intelligence and undeniable consciousness. They have an extensive vocabulary and are extremely affectionate. Yet every year millions of these animals are inhumanely raised and slaughtered to feed humans.

On numerous occasions people have said to me, "But meat tastes too good. I could never give it up." It saddens me to know that people cherish taste more than animal life.

If you want to learn more about the industry of factory farming, and the cruelty and exploitation of animals, I suggest watching a variety of documentaries (PETA, 2019). Refer to page 251 for a list of recommended films and other resources.

2) Health

One of the other biggest reasons people switch to a vegan diet is to become healthier. Numerous studies prove that eating a whole-food, plant-based diet is the healthiest approach.

According to the Academy of Nutrition and Dietetics, people who eat a plant-based diet are less likely to develop heart disease, cancer, diabetes or high blood pressure than meat-eaters.

People who eat a plant-based diet get all the nutrients that they need to be healthy, such as protein, fibre, vitamins, minerals and antioxidants without the cholesterol and saturated fat found in animal products, that depletes energy and increases risk of disease.

Much of the meat, dairy and eggs found in grocery stores come from factory farms that raise animals in sub-optimal conditions, resulting in sick animals. The steroids and antibiotics given to the animals, to manage or prevent infections, are passed on to humans when the meat is consumed. Eating plants prevents this.

According to research almost 70 percent of the North American population is overweight or obese due to poor diets and inactive lifestyles (Statistics Canada 2015). Experts have proven that a diet rich in plant-based foods, and daily activity, would positively impact these statistics dramatically.

If weight loss is one of your personal goals, converting to a whole-food, plant-based diet is the easiest way to shed those unwanted pounds, gain better health and reduce risk of disease.

When healthy changes are made weight management is a positive side effect that occurs with ease. A diet rich in plant-based foods provides the body with the essential nutrients it needs to run at its optimal capacity.

Imagine embracing a vegan lifestyle and in a short time you feel better than ever before. How would that make you feel?

Some of the positive benefits you will experience when eating a diet rich in whole, plant-based food include:

- Toxins are stored in fat cells to protect the body from harm. When the diet is clean and toxins are released from the body, it makes it easier to shed excess and unwanted weight.

- Reduced inflammation caused by high acid foods like animal products and processed foods resulting in less risk of developing a chronic disease.

- More energy.

- Better and more restful sleep.

- Healthier skin, nails, hair, teeth and gums.

- Enhanced mood and emotional health.

Refer to page 251 for a list of books and other resources that illustrate the health benefits of a plant-based diet.

3) Environment

Another popular reason people choose to shift to a whole-food, plant-based diet is to have a positive impact on the environment.

Raising animals for meat is not green. It's been said by scientific researchers that we cannot consider ourselves environmentalists if we still eat meat or other animal products (Science 2018).

According to PETA (2019), to produce one pound of beef it takes more than 2,400 gallons of water and 10 pounds of grain. To produce one pound of tofu it takes only 244 gallons of water and no grain.

The extra grain, and other plant food not eaten by these animals, can then be used to feed millions of hungry people around the world.

It is the opinion of environmental experts that consuming meat is one of the worst things we can do for the Earth. It is wasteful and causes enormous amounts of pollution.

Numerous sources state that the factory farming industry massively contributes to climate change.

According to the Humane Society of The United States (2019), in the U.S. alone, over 10 billion land animals are raised for dairy, meat and eggs. These animals contribute to 37 percent of methane emissions, which has 20 times the global warming effect of CO_2 .

These confined animals generate three times more raw waste materials than humans, which affect the water supply, ocean-life and contaminates the soil.

Adopting a plant-based diet is more effective than driving a "greener" car in the fight against climate change.

If you want to learn more about the effects of the agriculture industry to the environment refer to page 251 for a list of recommended documentaries and other resources.

Chapter 3:
11 Things You Need To Know Before Going Meatless

Making the choice to embrace a meatless lifestyle is one you will not regret. However, it is a huge life change and one you will not want to take lightly. There are many things to research and fully understand before making the switch to maintain good health.

1) Going Meatless Is A Personal Choice

Considering a meatless lifestyle is a very personal choice. It usually runs deeper than most people realize.

We have already discussed the three top reasons why people choose to go meatless and become vegan.

Others reasons include:

- **Culture or religion**. Many cultures and religions around the world advocate a vegan lifestyle for religious purposes.

- **Other people are doing it.** With a vegan lifestyle being one of the biggest movements in the world right now people see online influencers, celebrities and their social circle making the switch. This makes it easier to find inspiration and support from a broader community.

- **Can't tolerate eating meat anymore.** Often because the human body was not designed to process a lot of meat, since we are considered more herbivorous, or omnivorous at most, the body may one day find it hard to digest too much meat. Often, the more spiritual a person becomes the less meat they are able to eat. Meat is a heavy, dead food and it doesn't resonate with the lighter side of spiritual energy.

- **Meatless food is delicious.** Whether or not a person decides to go meatless they can't deny that plant-based food is absolutely amazing. Some of the best restaurants I have eaten at are vegan. I've had people come to my cooking classes, or home for dinner, unsure of what to expect and leave impressed by the delicious meal.

Regardless of your motivation to make the switch to a meatless lifestyle, believe in yourself and stay true to your decision. This will protect and keep you strong when others place judgment on your choice.

2) Prepare To Face Judgement From Others

Deciding to go meatless will bring positive change to your life. However, with change often comes fear. You may be confident in your decision but feel doubt and judgement when questioned by other people.

This is normal. People will always resist and fear change. The question is, how do you deal with this judgment in a way that will respect both you and your loved ones?

Here are a few tips:

a) Understand and empathize with their points of view.

They probably don't know why you've decided to go meatless because they're not yet educated on the benefits of this lifestyle.

When they ask questions about your motives ask them why they feel going meatless is a bad decision. They may have a belief about the lifestyle that's holding them back and you can help to educate them and relieve their worries.

Ask if you can share your reasons and offer some educational information on the benefits. Avoid telling them that their point of view is stupid or judging them on their choices.

If you want people to be understanding of your decisions you must pay them the same respect.

35

b) Never take things personally.

You've made a decision to change your entire lifestyle, which was likely, not an easy decision to make. However, your choice has deep meaning for you and that's all that matters.

People may say hurtful things, such as, "I could never go meatless because I love bacon," or, "animals are stupid so they don't deserve to live anyway" (yes, I've heard that one). But, they say it because they don't have the information you do and are not yet aware of the many benefits of a meatless lifestyle.

Just remember, their comments are coming from their lack of understanding, inner fear and ignorance. It has nothing to do with you and is none of your business. Just let what they say roll off your back and love them anyway.

c) Love them where they are now.

Unless you were one of the lucky ones whose parents raised you meatless, at one point you also ate and used animal products. Which means you were once where they are now.

The best thing you can do, if you want people to support your choices, is to love them for where they are now and stay true to yourself. By simply being who you are, living your lifestyle, without judgment or preaching, you will inspire people to make changes in their own lives.

3) There Is A Lot To Learn

Much confusion and misinformation exists around living a meatless lifestyle. Some will say it is the healthiest way to live, while others say it's not. A diet rich in plant-based food has been shown to be one of the healthiest way to eat. However, it's important to know how to do it correctly or, like any diet, it can be very unhealthy.

What do many people do when they decide to go meatless? They often turn to a diet filled with processed junk food. Just because the package says vegan does not mean it's healthy.

Many people who become vegan forget that "veg" is in the word. I have spoken to many vegetarians and vegans who don't even eat vegetables! They consume only processed pasta, breads and packaged junk food and wonder why they're sick and gaining weight.

To be a healthy vegan you must do your research and understand what nutrients you need to include in your diet. Better yet consult with a health professional who is trained in plant-based diets.

To be a healthy vegan some key things to consider are:

a) Eat an abundance of fresh fruits and vegetables

Yes, you must eat fresh produce to be healthy. According to the revised Canada Food Guide (Government of Canada 2019), for optimal health half of the diet must be rich in fruits and vegetables and the other half as whole-grains and protein. Eating this much fresh produce can be difficult for some people but it can be done. You can have fresh produce washed, cut, and ready to eat at all times. Smoothies are an easy way to blend up a delicious mix of fruits and vegetables. If you still feel you need extra, you can take a whole-food supplement to bridge the gap between what you're eating and what you should be eating.

b) Eat omega fatty acids

A good balance of omegas are essential for brain and overall healthy body function. Plant-based sources of omega fatty acids include hemp seeds, chia seeds, pumpkin seeds, flax seeds and blue-green algae. If you find you cannot eat enough of these foods then I suggest investing in a supplement that is rich in high-quality plant-based omegas.

c) Take a vitamin B12

Vitamin B12 is required for proper red blood cell formation, neurological function and DNA synthesis. Vegans don't usually get enough vitamin B12 because it comes from bacteria found on meat and fermented foods. To get enough of this vitamin eat fortified food, fermented food or take a supplement.

There is more to becoming vegan than just cutting out meat. It's important to do your homework and learn as much as you can from a professional and credible source before you get started to make sure you maintain optimal health.

To gain more information on this subject you may choose to:

a) Get help

Receiving help from a certified and credible professional is a great step to making the switch in a healthy way. Knowing how to eat a well-balanced, nutritionally dense diet will set you up for success.

Today, there are more educated professionals than ever before experienced in helping people with plant-based nutrition. Do your research and find someone in your area you can trust and learn from.

b) Read books, articles and blogs

Many books, articles and blogs exist to help you transition to a plant-based diet and educate you about the benefits of adopting this lifestyle. A simple internet search will lead you to a variety of great resources.

A word of caution: although we can learn a lot from someone's personal experience it's also important to know the educational background of the person you are learning from. Always be sure you are getting your information from a credible source.

c) Watch documentaries

Documentaries, movies and other videos will provide you with more knowledge and greater confidence in your decision. However, just like books, articles and blogs you can learn a lot from a documentary but be sure to base your health decisions on advice from qualified health professionals.

d) Take a course

A great way to learn more is to take a course or program that specializes in plant-based nutrition.

Please visit my website to learn more about my signature programs and other ways I can help you on this exciting journey.

4) It's Not Always Going To Be Easy

Picture this...

You've decided to transition to a vegan lifestyle and you're excited about it. You're expanding your knowledge and learning about what foods to eat and what companies test on animal or use their products.

Then you realize one of your favourite foods has dairy in it, your favourite line of shoes is only available in leather, your favourite hair care line tests on animals or your best friend loves to eat bacon everyday.

Then it hits you. You're a vegan living in a non-vegan world. Everywhere you look you realize animals are exploited and used in many products. Soon, your friends start to give you a hard time about your lifestyle and some even leave your life saying that you have changed too much and you're now too different.

Believe it or not, this is normal. It happens to all of us. Although being vegan is one of the most selfless and compassionate choices you can make, it will not always be easy.

However, how you look at it will make the difference. If your reasons for going meatless are clear it will be easier to deal with resistance from the outside world.

To make the switch to a meatless lifestyle a little easier, follow these simple steps:

a) Know your reasons with 100 percent conviction. That way no matter what anyone says you can always feel confident in your choice.

b) Go easy on yourself. You don't always have to be perfect. No one is. If you feel you've gone against your beliefs and consumed or used a non-vegan product, just take note, forgive yourself, bless the animal and continue to do your best.

c) Take things slowly. One-step-at-a-time will get you to where you want to go.

d) If your friends leave your life because you have chosen to go meatless then they likely were never true friends. This is a perfect time to develop a new community of like-minded people.

5) You Are Part Of A Growing Community

Going meatless has been shown to be one of the biggest lifestyle movements today.

A new poll commissioned by the Vancouver Humane Society (2015) shows that 33 percent of Canadians, or almost 12 million, are either already vegetarian or are eating less meat.

In the United States, about 16 million people are vegetarian and about half of those are vegan. This means you are part of a growing community and have a lot of support.

Many cities have local meet-up groups, restaurants and communities that support and celebrate the vegan lifestyle. Search your local community for an opportunity to connect with like-minded people so you feel supported, free to be yourself and learn from others' experiences.

Many local and international speakers educate on the topic. Search the Internet for events and social media platforms for groups and experts to follow.

6) Be Prepared To Answer Dumb Questions

I say dumb in the nicest way possible because truthfully there are no dumb questions, just inquiries. The reason vegans get asked so many questions is because people don't know what it means to be vegan or understand why anyone would choose to live this way.

Many new vegans get angry and defensive when people ask them questions about being vegan. I know I did when I first made the switch. However, I encourage you to welcome all questions as an opportunity to educate an inquiring mind.

These questions may seem silly to you now but you were once where they are now. Besides, you never know, your answer might inspire them to join you on your new mission. If you answer defensively, or get annoyed, you might turn them off of the lifestyle forever.

Here's a list of some of the common questions vegans are asked:

a) Where do you get your protein?

This is probably the question vegans are asked the most. The thing about this question is that it's a prime opportunity to educate people about nutrition.

Protein is in every living cell, which means any whole food, whether it's animal or plant-based, contains protein.

Many people worry that eating a plant-based diet won't provide enough protein. However, this is far from the truth. Many plant-based foods not only contain protein but many are complete proteins.

A complete protein is a food source of protein that contains an adequate proportion of each of the nine essential amino acids necessary in the human diet.

Complete protein foods include:

- Soy
- Quinoa
- Buckwheat
- A combination of rice and beans (two incomplete proteins make a complete protein)

An incomplete protein source is one that may be low in, or lacking one or more, essential amino acids.

Sources of incomplete protein foods include:

- Beans
- Lentils
- Nuts
- Seeds
- Dark leafy greens

Plant-based foods require less energy for the body to digest than animal protein and the nutrients are easily absorbed.

The main issue with this question is that while everyone is concerned about getting enough protein they are eliminating complex carbohydrates and lacking in the fibre and nutrients these foods provide.

However, according to nutrition sciences, an active person requires six to 10 grams of carbohydrates per kilogram of bodyweight and only 0.8 to 1.7 grams of protein per kilogram of bodyweight (American Council on Exercise (2014).

Carbohydrates and fibre are critical in supporting healthy digestion and reducing risk of various chronic diseases (Campbell & Campbell 2006).
Which makes me question why people are so concerned about protein intake when carbohydrates are the body's preferred fuel source.

b) Isn't it hard to be vegan?

This is a question I find funny now. It's so easy to be vegan that non-vegans can hardly comprehend the simplicity of it. It's much easier to make a quick salad than prepare a steak dinner.

Many cookbooks, and online blogs, are readily available and have easy-to-make and delicious recipes that support a smooth transition.

If you are new to eating plant-based food the key is to go easy on yourself. You may not be perfect all the time but by doing the best you can you are enhancing your health, saving the animals and reducing your impact on the earth.

c) "Don't you miss the taste of meat?"

This question is usually followed by, "I could never give up meat. I like the taste of it too much."

For those of us who really love animals this question can make our hearts ache because we could never imagine hurting an animal just to taste their meat. In this situation, avoid the temptation to go into a long speech about animal cruelty. This will only make things worse.

Simply respond by letting the person know that there are many delicious meat alternatives available on the market. I know I have made these meat alternative options for many friends and family who haven't even noticed the difference.

Some of my favourite "meatless" food brands include:

- **Gardein™**: Offers a variety of meatless alternatives such as the beefless burger, meatless meatballs, chick'n sliders and nuggets, turk'y cutlets and fish sticks.

- **Beyond Meat™**: Offers the famous beyond burger, which has gone global at A&W™. They also make sausages, which are so close to the real meat version, that some people have a hard time believing it's not real meat. The first time I tried the beyond burger it was too similar to meat that I couldn't eat it.

- **Tofurkey™**: Offers meatless sausages, veggie burgers, deli slices, a meat-free ham and stuffed turkey-like roast.

- **Follow Your Heart™**: Offers vegan mayonnaise, vegan cheese, salad dressings and egg replacer.

- **Daiya™**: Offers vegan shredded cheese, cream cheese, cheezy mac™ and burritos.

d) "What would happen to all the animals if we stopped eating them?"

The entire world would not become vegan overnight so in time the numbers of animals raised for food would slowly decline.

As the number of factory farms and farm animals decline and the destruction of land and rainforests for farming decreases, wildlife populations would recover.

In her podcast episode, Colleen Patrick Goudreau (2016) talks about this very question. She says that animals raised for food are genetic abominations and are best left to go extinct. These animals have been bred to be bigger and fatter than they would naturally. They suffer illness and great stress to their skeletal system from their unnatural large body size.

e) "What's wrong with eggs and dairy? Those animals don't have to be slaughtered."

Although it is true these animals are kept alive in order to collect their products, the living conditions for them are often inhumane. Cows are artificially inseminated and their babies are ripped away from them as soon as they are born so their milk can be collected. This means the babies are shipped off to small crates to be raised for veal or slaughtered.

Chickens are kept in small cages, or if they're "free-range" they still don't have much room to move since there are thousands of chickens in one barn.

When baby chicks are born they are separated by gender. The females are kept to lay eggs and the males are thrown in the garbage or ground up alive and fed to other animals.

f) "Why don't vegans eat honey? Bees are not factory farmed or slaughtered."

This is true. Bees are not factory farmed like cows, chickens or pigs but they can suffer when honey and pollen are taken from their hives.

Honey is the energy source, or food, for bees. According to The Vegan Society (2019), when conventional honey farmers remove the honey they replace it with a sugar substitute, which is bad for the bees health. Also, bees are bred to increase production, which narrows the gene pool and increases risk of disease and depletion of bee populations on a large scale.

Bees will often have their wings clipped to prevent them from leaving the hive and honey collection machines often crush the bees or slice them in half leaving them to suffer.

If you meet a vegan who eats honey they likely buy from a local farmer who uses humane techniques where the bees are raised in a healthy manner and not harmed during honey collection and production.

7) You Will Help Save The Earth

One main reason why people choose to become vegan is environmental.

As you learned in chapter two, because of the mass destruction of the planet for agricultural business, you cannot consider yourself an environmentalist if you still eat meat or other animal products. Meat is not green.

Beautiful Mother Earth is our home. She provides us with water, food, shelter and beauty for us to enjoy. When you develop a connection to the planet you feel a sense of peace and connection to yourself and to spirit.

All living things on this planet are here for a reason. While we're here, let's do a better job of protecting this beautiful planet for generations to come. It starts with us choosing to only support companies that follow conscious and compassionate business practices.

8) Eat Whole Foods Not Just Vegan Junk Food

It can be tempting when you first go meatless to eat all the junk food you can find. Yes, there are many delicious treats that are vegan. However; they are just that. Treats to be enjoyed on occasion.

A meatless lifestyle is the best way to gain optimal health but only if you are eating whole food and not just replacing animal food with processed food.

As a new vegan, you may be tempted to trade in meat for bread and pasta thinking you are doing a good thing. However, you are only setting yourself up for failure. To be a healthy vegan your diet must consist of a variety of whole, unprocessed foods

50

including fresh fruits and vegetables, beans, nuts and seeds.

There are too many vegans who eat nothing but processed bread, pasta and vegan junk food. They are unhealthy and give veganism a bad name. When all they eat is junk food it's no wonder people think being vegan is unhealthy. Any diet is unhealthy if it consists of mostly highly processed, sugary foods and low in essential nutrients.

In saying this, there is nothing wrong with having a treat every once in awhile.

Find a vegan cookbook or search for delicious recipes online. Some of your traditional favourite treats and meals can be easily transformed into healthy vegan alternatives.

Be an advocate for the vegan community. Take care of your health, be a role model and inspire others to upgrade their health with a whole-food, vegan lifestyle.

9) It's Okay To Take It Slowly

Choosing to become vegan is a different experience for everyone. Some people watch a documentary that awakens them to the horrors of factory farming and stop eating animals immediately.

Others, like me, take their time and slowly cut out animal products as they learn more about how to do it in a healthy way.

Regardless of why or how you choose to go meatless, the important thing is that you are doing it.

When going meatless, be kind to others who are learning how to adopt this new lifestyle. Encourage people to do the best they can and educate, rather than judge them, because they may not be perfect right away.

If, once you choose to go meatless, you accidentally, or even purposefully, consume animal products, is it the end of the world? No. The best thing to do is be kind to yourself, recognize how it makes you feel and think about how you can avoid consuming it in the future.

It's not about being perfect. It's about doing your best because every little bit counts. One of the biggest reasons many people refuse a meatless lifestyle is because there are so many die-hard vegans in the world that will judge anyone who even thinks about eating animals or using an animal product. Rather than inspire people by being a role model who is filled with love and compassion for themselves and others.

I have to admit, when I first became vegan I was a bit like that and got into arguments over it. I was so distraught over the animal cruelty I witnessed online.

I was also shocked to learn the many detrimental health effects that results from eating animals that I couldn't wrap my head around why anyone could still eat these foods.

However; I quickly learned that judging people for their choices is no way to educate and inspire them to make the switch. I am not perfect and it's not necessary for anyone else to be. Those of us who decide to become vegan need to simply focus on why we chose this lifestyle and stay true to ourselves. When we do, we are more likely to inspire someone else to make better choices.

10) You Must Supplement Your Diet

As a vegan it's important to supplement your diet with some nutrients you may not be able to get from food alone. However, it's important to speak with a qualified health professional before consuming any synthetic supplements as many supplements on the market are not regulated and can, and often do, cause more harm than good.

Whole-food supplementation is important in any diet for a few reasons:

- The produce we buy in stores has lost at least 50 percent of its nutritional value from when it leaves the field to when we buy and eat it.

- The quality of the soil the produce is grown in is poor; therefore, the food has low nutritional value.

- It is not always possible to eat enough food for optimal health.

- Some nutrients are more difficult to get from plants.

The one main supplement recommended for vegans specifically is vitamin B12. Other suggested supplements are mentioned in chapter eight.

11) You Will Get Enough Protein On A Vegan Diet

The misconception around the fact that a vegan diet does not provide a person, including high-level athletes, with enough protein is easily dispelled with science.

The China Study (Campbell & Campbell, 2006), compares a variety of nutrients of plant-based foods (equal parts of tomatoes, spinach, lima beans, peas and potatoes) to animal-based foods (equal parts of beef, pork, chicken and whole milk).

The results clearly show that the nutrient density of plant-based foods is far superior. This means plant-based foods provide the body with more healing nutrients than animal products.

In the chart below, you will see that when compared to equal parts of animal-based foods, plant-based foods yield comparable amounts of protein (33 vs. 34 grams). This means that a diet rich in plant-based foods will provide adequate amounts of protein.

Nutrient Composition of Plant and Animal Based Foods (per 500 calories of energy) Source: The China Study by Dr. T. Colin Campbell, Thomas M. Campbell II (May 11/06)		
Nutrient	**Plant-Based Foods**	**Animal-Based Foods**
Cholesterol (mg)	---	137
Fat (g)	4	36
Protein (g)	33	34
Beta-carotene (mcg)	29,919	17
Dietary Fiber (g)	31	---
Vitamin C (mg)	293	4
Folate (mcg)	1168	19
Vitamin E (mg_ATE)	11	0.5
Iron (mg)	20	2
Magnesium (mg)	548	51
Calcium (mg)	545	252

A BEGINNERS GUIDE TO GOING MEATLESS

Chapter 4:
Simple Steps To Going Meatless

If you're still reading this book you must be ready to become meatless. Congratulations! You are about to embark on an exciting journey.

In this chapter, I will review simple steps you can take right now to make this change a little easier and long lasting.

Before we get into these steps let me share a story.

One day I was getting together with a friend of mine who couldn't wrap his head around the fact that I was now vegan. This is someone I used to eat steak and drink red wine with on a fairly regular basis. He is an avid meat eater and said he couldn't imagine not eating his favourite foods.

One day we were enjoying a glass of wine before eating a beautiful meal his wife prepared for us, when he asked, "now that you're vegan what can you eat?"

I smiled, knowing that he was struggling to figure out my new way of eating, and asked him to look at it from a different perspective.

I encouraged him to look at the abundance of food we were about to enjoy together.

Then I challenged him to think about what would be left if we were to take away all the plant foods on the table including the spices, cooking oils and most of the side dishes.

He looked at me knowing I was right. If we took away the plants all that would be left would be a bland roast beef. At that moment he got it.

Even a meat eater will eat plant-based foods at some point. For optimal health it's essential that everyone, vegan or not, eat over half of their diet in whole, plant-based foods. It's these fresh vitamin and mineral rich foods that keep us healthy and allow the body to thrive. No one can be healthy by eating meat alone.

He nodded and agreed. Of course, he still had to defend his position, reiterate that he could never give up his meat and stuffed a big piece of beef in his mouth.

The point is, that as a vegan you will not be deprived. You have an abundance of food options that you may not even know about yet.

If you are ready to get started then follow these simple steps and you will be well on your way to transforming your life, saving animals and sustaining the planet.

1) Start With One Meal, Or One Day Per Week

If all you did to start was cut out animal products for one day, or even one meal per week, you would be making a huge difference to your health, animal life and the environment.

A study on the amount of greenhouse gas emissions resulting from diet choices showed that greenhouse gas emissions are twice as high for meat eaters than vegans (Scarborough et al. (2014).

According to Environmental Defence, if one person skipped a meal of chicken per week and substituted this meal with plant-based foods, the reduction in CO_2 would be the same as taking more than half a million cars off the road (Freston, 2011). That's a pretty significant impact with just one simple step!

2) Eliminate Processed Meats

Processed meats, whether you're meatless or not, have no place in a healthy diet. These include any cured meats such as bacon, hotdogs and deli meats such as bologna and salami.

According to the World Health Organization these meats are particularly harmful to your health and contribute to a variety of diseases such as heart disease and cancer (American Cancer Society, 2015).

If you did nothing else but stop eating processed meat, you'd be positively impacting your health. If you really miss these meats there are a variety of plant-based options such as meat-free deli slices and sausages now available in your local grocery store.

2) Eliminate Red Meat And Pork

Red meat and pork have been shown to be leading contributors to disease due to the high content of saturated fat (American Heart Association, 2015).

If you find it hard to eliminate these meats for health reasons, then I suggest looking at the hard reality of what these animals go through in factory farms. If you have a compassionate heart you won't be able to watch the cruel treatment and contribute to it any longer. It will give you a good solid reason to cut it out for good.

3) Eliminate Poultry

Poultry includes chicken, turkey and any other birds. Many people think chicken is healthy food. However, it couldn't be further from the truth. Studies have shown that poultry often contains arsenic and steroids that have been injected into the bird to make it grow and prevent illness from the poor living conditions. As a result of all of this, commercial chicken is rife with salmonella, feces and toxic pollutants (Greger, 2019).

Another study found that bacterium in poultry may be responsible for causing chronic bladder infections in humans (Science Daily, 2018).

If you find it hard to eliminate poultry for health reasons, watch videos of the cruel treatment these animals endure and ask yourself if you want to continue to contribute to their suffering.

4) Eliminate Fish And Other Seafood

Fish is also considered a healthy food in the mainstream nutrition community. However, due to contaminants in fish, it's not something you want to be eating for optimal health (Clement, 2014).

Although fish has healthy fats like omegas, there are many healthier plant alternatives such as blue-green algae. Most of the wild fish in our oceans are contaminated by radiation and pollution and farmed fish are often sick and full of lice from swimming in their own excrement and overpopulation in tanks.

Consider this, to catch a fish they are either caught in a large net, where many whales, dolphins, turtles and other sea life are accidentally killed, or on a hook. These animals are then brought out of their environment and left to suffocate until they die.

Shellfish, like crab and lobster, feel pain as much as any other animal, yet have their limbs pulled from them and are boiled alive.

5) Eliminate Dairy And Eggs

Dairy and eggs seem to be the hardest for people to eliminated from the diet. Most people believe these products are okay to eat since the animal is not killed. However, this is untrue. These animals suffer greatly so humans can take these products to eat.

Dairy products are made from the milk a female cow produces when she gives birth to feed her calf. These cows are usually artificially inseminated and the calf removed before it can drink the milk.

We are the only species on earth that consumes milk past infancy and consume another species' milk.

Dairy causes high levels of inflammation in the body, which places us at greater risk of disease. The dairy industry has told the general population that milk "does a body good" and that it's a good source of calcium. However, it has been shown that people who consume high amounts of dairy have the highest rates of osteoporosis and other chronic illnesses (Greger, 2017).

Eggs are the reproductive secretions of chickens and are often thought to be a good source of protein. However, Dr. Michael Greger has reviewed studies that show a strong link between breast and prostate cancer and egg consumption (Greger, 2019).

6) Replace Animal Products With Plant-Based Options

You can easily replace meat with plant-based options such as:

- Beans
- Lentils
- Tofu
- Tempeh
- Seitan
- Nuts
- Mushrooms
- Plant-based meat-like products

For example, if making chilli or tacos use beans, mushrooms or Gardein Beefless Ground™, instead of beef or chicken.

In baking, eggs can be replaced with pureed bananas, ground chia or ground flax seeds mixed with water. The best part about using these replacements is that you can eat the raw cookie dough and not have to worry about getting salmonella from raw eggs.

Nuts make a delicious cheese and many plant-based cheese options are available for purchase in your local natural food store.

Cow's milk is an easy one to replace, as there are many dairy-free varieties including, nuts, hemp, soy, rice and coconut.

Use a nut-base or commercial vegan cheese in place of dairy cheese for your grilled cheese sandwich or pizza.

7) Make Half Your Diet Rich In Fruits And Vegetables

The new Canada Food Guide (2019) recommends that over half of the diet should consist of whole fruits and vegetables. The good news is, once you begin your transition to becoming vegan you will notice how much more food there is to eat. When you're eating lighter, more nutrient dense foods, as opposed to heavy meat-based meals rich in saturated fat, you will feel lighter and able to eat more.

For best results, eat as much variety as you can. If you're not a big fan of eating vegetables because you don't like the taste, then you must train your taste buds to like these new foods.

It's no different than training the muscles of the body to be stronger or to have more endurance. Your taste buds get used to the foods you eat and must be trained to enjoy new ones that don't contain as much salt, sugar and fat.

Start this taste-bud-training process by eating a new vegetable or fruit each week. You may be surprised by how delicious these foods are when you prepare and cook them in creative ways.

8) Eat Legumes Daily

Legumes include beans, lentils and peas. These foods are rich in healthy carbohydrates, fibre, protein, vitamins and minerals. Studies have shown that increasing the daily intake of legumes can prevent a variety of chronic diseases (Greger, 2019).

Many varieties of legumes exist. So, try them all. Be creative and make new recipes by combining them with different ingredients to determine which ones you like best.

9) Eat Nuts And Seeds Daily

Nuts and seeds contain healthy fats, fibre and protein that will help the body gain better health and fight disease. Dr. Greger (2019), and other nutrition experts, suggest that eating even just a quarter cup of nuts or seeds each day can help enhance health and reduce risk of disease.

Nuts are best eaten in their raw, unsalted form. Nuts that are lower in fat, like almonds, are best soaked in filtered water for two to six hours before eating to awaken enzymes that help with digestion and encourage better nutrient absorption.

10) Search For New Recipes And Be Creative

Numerous websites, blogs and books exist to showcase an abundance of delicious plant-based recipes. Find a favourite and get cooking.

Visit my website: **www.LivingMeatless.com/recipes** or make the recipes included in this book to get started.

11) Have Quick And Easy Meals Handy

Keep pre-packaged meals, such as veggie burgers, plant-based meats, pizza and other quick options handy when you are short on time. Make big batches of food, such as a large pot of spaghetti, a pan of lasagna, a large pot of soup or a batch of chilli. Freeze these meals in single or family serving size containers and pull out each dish when you're ready to eat.

12) Eat Ethnic Foods

Ethnic cuisine, such as Indian, Middle Eastern and Asian, are often meat and dairy-free and full of flavour. However, before ordering one of these dishes in a restaurant be sure to confirm that they do not use dairy, fish sauce or other animal-based ingredients in their recipes.

13) Seek Out Vegan-Friendly Restaurants

Endless options exist when it comes to eating plant-based meals in restaurants. Many mainstream restaurants are now offering meatless options on the menu making it much easier to be social with people who still choose to eat meat.

Where I live there is vegan Indian, Chinese, Thai and Vietnamese cuisine. I'm sure you can find the same, if not more, options in your area.

What I love the most about eating at vegan restaurants is they are often more health and environmentally conscious and use local and fresh ingredients to create mouth-watering meals.

14) Look In Your Cupboards

Chances are you already have more meatless food in your kitchen than you thought. Remember, anything that isn't meat, dairy or egg is vegan.

Foods such as beans, rice, pasta, peanut butter, cereal, fruit and vegetables are plant-based and are likely in your cupboards, or fridge, right now.

15) Shop At Your Local Grocery Store

Take a look around your local grocery store. It used to be that you'd have to shop at a specialized natural food store to find vegan options, outside of fruits and vegetables, but now even local grocery stores carry plant-based options such as dairy-free milk and meat-free dinner options.

If you are unsure of an ingredient ask the staff.

16) Do Your Research

Read books, articles and blogs from plant-based experts, watch documentaries and connect with people in your community to learn as much as you can about eating a meatless diet.

Many professionals are now doing this work. Seek out new resources and make this a continual learning and growing experience to help you become a healthier, happier and more conscious consumer.

The more you learn about the benefits of a plant-based lifestyle, and connect with people who have the same values as you, the easier it will be to maintain your new lifestyle.

17) Take It One Step At A Time

If you want to develop healthier habits, write down all the unhealthy habits you would like to convert into healthier ones. Once you have this list, choose one to work with.

For example, let's say you want to quit smoking, quit drinking, eat better, drink more water and exercise more. It would be a disaster if you tried to change all of these habits at once. Instead, you will be more successful if you start with one habit to change, such as drinking more water, master that one then choose another.

Yes, some people can adopt a meatless lifestyle overnight. However, for the majority, taking it one-step-at-a-time will result in better success.

18) Be Kind To Yourself And Others

Being kind to yourself when making this, or any other changes in your life, is critical to success.

Give yourself a break from judgment and criticism and replace these thoughts and feelings with love and compassion. You are human and bound to make mistakes. It's all part of the journey.

If you choose to go meatless but mess up and eat dairy chocolate or some other animal-based treat, rather than beating yourself up, just forgive yourself and move on.

Besides, the more you love yourself the easier it is to make positive changes.

Being kind to others is also extremely important. If you have chosen to be vegan then it's your responsibility to live the compassionate lifestyle it is meant to be.

Many of us choose to be vegan because we can't stand the cruelty that happens to animals in factory farming or the destruction of the environment. Therefore, if we want to change this world we must be the change we want to see.

This means sending love and compassion to the people in your life who don't understand your choice. Love them where they are at now and remember that at one point you were there too.

Be kind to people who are working hard to become vegan but "mess up" every once in awhile. This lifestyle is not about perfection; it's about doing the best we can. Support the people who are struggling to make this big change, even if that person is you. Forgive, understand and send them love and support. It's this positive energy that helps inspire success.

Send love and compassion to people who work in factory farms and who are responsible for the horrific acts that take place towards animals and the environment.

I understand it's not easy to send love to people who cause unbelievable pain, destruction and suffering. However; I believe the positive energy we give to the people in this world, whether we know them or not, will impact them in some way. Therefore, do your best to be a role model and live as a loving and compassionate person at all times.

Chapter 5:
What Is Whole Food?

You have likely heard the term whole food before. I'm sure you know that eating a diet rich in healthy food is better for you and will reduce your risk of disease. But what does healthy, whole-food, actually mean? Why is it important to eat a diet rich in whole-food?

Whole foods are fruits and vegetables, legumes, whole grains and nuts that are unaltered and remain in their original form. These foods have been grown from the earth, picked and eaten in their natural form. Once any food has been modified it is no longer considered a true whole food.

For example, many people believe whole-grain bread or pasta is a whole food. Unfortunately, since the ingredients that make up these foods are no longer in their natural state they are considered a processed food and should be consumed only on occasion.

Since the beginning of time our Mother Earth has provided us with natural, healing nutrients including herbs people have used as medicine for centuries. Unfortunately, since the rise of the pharmaceutical

71

industry many of these methods of natural healing have been abandoned.

However, the good news is, we are starting to become aware of these ancient methods and realize that all we need to do to obtain optimal health and heal ourselves is with the food Mother Earth provides.

The Standard American Diet is plagued with food full of saturated fat, sugar and salt, which wreak havoc on our internal organs and emotional health (Imatome-Yun, 2016).

In our grab-and-go society, we have become accustomed to eating food in pretty little packages. Little concern is given to the fact that these processed, packaged foods are laden with chemicals and lacking the nutrition our body needs to function properly.

A diet lacking in essential nutrients results in overeating, weight gain, obesity and other health problems including diabetes, heart disease and cancer.

This Standard American Diet, consisting mostly of processed foods, red and processed meats, poultry, high fat dairy products and highly refined, sugary foods, has been shown to result in higher risk of disease.

Even the World Health Organization has recognized that processed meats negatively impact health and encourages people to cut down on the consumption of these foods (American Cancer Society, 2015).

A diet rich in animal-based and processed foods and low in fruits and vegetables, results in an acidic state causing inflammation. This inflammation leads to disease, pain and suffering. Your body can only be healthy if it is in a non-acid state (Greger, 2019).

The pH Balance

Your blood is measured in terms of acidity or alkalinity, which is also known as the pH balance. A pH less than 7.0 is acidic and a pH higher than 7 is alkaline. Keeping a balanced internal environment in the body is important and necessary for optimal health.

The ideal pH for the blood is 7.4. Anything below or above this range results in symptoms of disease. Death can occur when pH is below 6.8 or above 7.8 (Schwalfenberg, 2012).

When you eat alkaline and nutrient-rich foods, such as raw fruits and vegetables, the body will detox and clean out toxins that have been stored in your tissues for years. This may result in flu-like symptoms, low energy levels, and a ride on the emotional rollercoaster. However; these symptoms will subside in only a few days leaving you feeling refreshed and full of energy.

Diets rich in raw, alkaline food have been shown to reverse the effects of long-term illness. Dr. Brian Clement, Director of the Hippocrates Health Institute in West Palm Beach, Florida, suggests that it may take one month to cleanse and repair for every year your body was exposed to poisonous foods and other toxins. That isn't too bad considering how many years your body has been exposed to potentially harmful toxins.

The body is an amazing machine and it transforms itself based on the foods you eat, what you put on your skin and breath through your lungs.

Every seven years your cellular tissue will completely renew and every 10 years your skeleton will be a new structure. This is often why we don't see chronic health issues appearing until later in life or after many years of toxic exposure. The time needed for the body to change at a cellular level is also why noticeable healthy changes will take months or even years to show on the outside.

This means that based on what you have eaten and been exposed to is how your body will respond and change. Therefore, you really are what you eat.

Alkaline & Acid Rich Foods

Raw, living food is considered to be the most nutritious food because the vitamins, minerals, enzymes and other nutrients have not been destroyed by heat or other processing methods.

When food is cooked at high temperatures, over 46° Celsius (115° Fahrenheit), precious enzymes and nutrients are destroyed and can no longer be used to heal or fuel the body. Therefore, it is critical to eat as much raw, living food as possible.

For best health, aim to consume alkaline-rich, raw, whole foods at least 80 percent of your diet and eat cooked, not-so-healthy foods the other 20 percent.

High To Low Alkaline Foods:

High Alkaline Foods:
- Broccoli
- Celery
- Dried figs
- Garlic
- Green herbs
- Herbal tea
- Lemon
- Parsley
- Spinach
- Sprouts
- Stevia
- Vegetable juice
- Watermelon
- Wheatgrass

Alkaline Foods:
- Almonds
- Apples
- Beets (raw)
- Berries
- Black currants
- Carrots
- Dates
- Grapes
- Green beans
- Green tea
- Hazelnuts
- Human breast milk
- Kiwi
- Kombucha
- Lima beans
- Lettuce
- Maple syrup
- Papaya
- Pears
- Rice syrup
- Zucchini

Low Alkaline Foods:

- Amaranth
- Asparagus
- Avocados
- Beets (cooked)
- Brazil nuts
- Buckwheat
- Cabbage
- Cauliflower
- Cherries
- Chestnuts
- Coconut
- Corn
- Flax seed oil
- Ginger tea
- Grapefruit
- Lentils
- Mangoes
- Millet
- Mushrooms
- Olives
- Onions
- Oranges
- Peaches
- Peas
- Pineapple
- Potatoes
- Quinoa
- Raisins
- Raw sugar
- Rhubarb
- Sour cherries
- Soybeans
- Soy milk
- Squash
- Strawberries
- Sunflower oil
- Tofu Soy cheese
- Tomatoes
- Turnip
- Wild rice

Low Acid Foods:

- Bananas
- Blueberries
- Brown rice
- Cocoa
- Cranberries
- Kidney beans
- Oats
- Plums
- Processed fruit juices
- Pumpkin seeds
- Rye bread
- Sesame seeds
- Spinach
- Sunflower seeds
- Sweet potatoes
- White sugar
- Whole grain bread

Acid Foods:

- Biscuits
- Brown sugar
- Canned fruit
- Cashew

76

- Jam
- Ketchup
- Mayonnaise
- Molasses
- Mustard
- Navy beans
- Pasta
- Pastries
- Pecans
- Pinto beans
- Pistachio
- Soda
- Wine
- White rice
- White bread

High Acid Foods:

- Beer
- Black tea
- Coffee
- Liquor
- Peanuts
- Pickled vegetables
- Walnuts

Chapter 6:
Introduction To Nutrition

An abundance of research has been done about nutrition and how the body uses the food we eat. Yet, there is still controversy and varying opinions about which diet is best for humans. However, if you look at the real science behind nutrition and stick to the basics it isn't that hard to see which diet is best.

Numerous studies have shown that the best diet for humans is one rich in whole food nutrients. This includes daily small to moderate portion sizes of fruits, vegetables, nuts, seeds, whole grains and legumes.

Sadly, with the invention of processed convenience foods and excessive portion sizes, the world's obesity and health problems have skyrocketed over the past few decades. Obesity Canada (2019) reports that over 30 percent of Canadians are obese. This extreme body fat results in chronic conditions that may require medical attention to manage.

Obesity is the leading cause of chronic diseases such as type II diabetes, high blood pressure, heart disease, stroke and cancer. It is said that one in 10 premature deaths in people ages 20 to 64 is the result of obesity (Obesity Canada, 2019).

It has come to the point where so many people are overweight and sick because of their diet, and other lifestyle choices, that individuals and governments cannot afford to keep up. The Canadian government projects that obesity related health-care costs will rise to over $9 billion by the year 2021 (Obesity Canada, 2019). This needs to change and it can.

Each one of us can make decisions every day that will either improve or negatively impact our health. This starts with the diet. It's important to choose whole foods rich in the right amount of macronutrients and micronutrients.

What Are Macronutrients?

Macronutrients include protein, carbohydrates and fats. These make up the food we eat that our body requires for fuel and recovery. Once ingested, the body breaks down protein to amino acids, carbohydrates to monosaccharides and fat to fatty acids. These chemical components are then absorbed in the body and delivered to the cells to support vital functions.

Many different opinions exist on how many of these macronutrients we need for optimal health. For best results it's important to find the balance that works best for you and your goals.

1) Carbohydrates

Carbohydrates serve a variety of vital functions and are one of the most important macronutrients. Carbohydrates are the body's preferred source of energy (providing four calories per gram) and the only energy source for red blood cells and the brain. Carbohydrates, especially in a high-fibre form, also help support digestive health and manage cholesterol levels.

Without using too much science jargon about chemical structure, explained are the various kinds of carbohydrates, categorized into monosaccharides (made of carbon and water) and disaccharides (made of two monosaccharides).

The American Council on Exercise (2014) defines monosaccharides as:

A) **Glucose**, also known as dextrose, is the basic building block of most carbohydrates and is the most predominant natural sugar.

B) **Fructose**, or fruit sugar, is the sweetest and found in fruit.

C) **Galactose** is as sweet as glucose and often bound to glucose to form lactose.

The American Council on Exercise (2014) defines disaccharides as:

A) **Lactose** made of the link between galactose and

glucose and is the predominant sugar in milk.

B) **Maltose** is made of two glucose molecules and better known as malt sugar.

C) **Sucrose** is made of glucose and fructose and more commonly known as table sugar.

Unfortunately, when people think about carbohydrates, they most often think of candy, baked goods, bread, pasta, cereal and mostly refined, white or whole-wheat sources of carbohydrates.

These refined carbohydrates are usually full of sugar and chemical preservatives, which harm the body, break down tissues and organs, cause weight gain and other health problems. However, these are not the kinds of carbohydrates the body requires for fuel.

What the body uses for fuel are healthy carbohydrates that come from pure earth-grown sources.

The best sources of whole-food carbohydrates include:

- Whole grains such as oats, brown rice, millet, amaranth, buckwheat, wild, black and brown rice and quinoa. Quinoa, is a seed and considered a pseudo grain since it contains an abundance of fibre and healthy carbohydrates. But it's also a source of complete protein.

82

- Starchy vegetables such as sweet and white potatoes, corn and squash.
- Fruits of all kinds.

These healthy carbohydrates not only provide fuel for the body but also fibre for healthy digestion, all while keeping cholesterol at healthy levels. Without these foods in the short term, people begin to feel the negative effects such as low energy, brain fog and crankiness. In the long term, people increase their risk of constipation, increased cholesterol, heart disease and cancer.

Many people shy away from eating healthy carbohydrates such as fruit, or other whole-food carbohydrate sources due to the high sugar content. However, even though there is sugar in these foods it is a natural sugar that the body efficiently uses for energy. These foods also contain fibre and a variety of essential micronutrients, like vitamins and minerals that the body needs for energy, healthy digestion and optimal health.

Therefore, most people do not eat enough of the right kind of carbohydrates such as whole-food complex carbs found in whole-grains and vegetables. As a result, fibre intake is low and digestive problems, like constipation and colon cancer, are more common than ever.

Recommended Intake

According to Potgieter (2012) who reviewed the latest guidelines from the American College of Sport Nutrition, a person who participates in general activity, requires three to five grams of carbohydrates per kilogram of body weight. Whereas an athlete may require six to 10 grams of carbohydrates per kilogram of body weight.

A sedentary person, someone who does fewer than 30 minutes of activity less than three days per week, may only need one and a half grams of carbohydrates per kilogram of body weight.

This is often where carbohydrates get a bad rap. It's not the carbs that are bad; it's overconsumption and underutilization that's causing the problem.

Think of it this way.

Carbohydrates are like gas in the tank of your car. You need to have gas in the tank to drive your car but the amount of gas you need will depend on how much you drive. If you're going on a long drive, you'll need a full tank of gas. If your car stays parked in the garage, or you're travelling a short distance, you won't need as much gas.

The same this is true with carbohydrates. Athletes, and others who train their body at higher levels of intensity, need more energy from carbohydrates than a person who is sick and lying in bed.

Regardless of activity levels, it's recommended that carbohydrates, specifically whole grains and food high in fibre, make up 45 percent to 65 percent of your total diet to adequately fuel your body .

Depending on the resource, and your personal goals, these numbers may vary. Studies show that of this carbohydrate intake, 21 to 38 grams of fibre per day is optimal for most adults (The National Academies of Sciences Engineering Medicine, 2002).

The Glycemic Index

To determine which carbohydrates are the best to consume many professionals refer to the glycemic index (GI). This system assigns a value to foods based on how slowly or how quickly they increase blood glucose levels (Diabetes Canada, 2013). Also known as "blood sugar," blood glucose levels above normal are toxic and can cause diabetes, which left uncontrolled may result in loss of limbs, blindness, kidney failure and increased risk of cardiovascular disease (Kawakhito et al., 2009).

Foods low on the GI scale (55 or less) tend to release glucose slowly and steadily, tend to contain higher levels of fibre and support weight loss. Foods high on the GI scale (70 or more) release glucose rapidly, are usually higher in sugar, help with energy during and after exercise and offset hypoglycemia (low blood sugar levels).

Glycemic Index Food Guide (Diabetes Canada, 2013)

Choose food **low on the Glycemic Index (55 or less)** most often.

These include:

Breads:
- Mixed grain bread
- Spelt bread
- Sourdough bread
- Tortilla

Cereal:
- All-Bran™ cereal
- All-Bran™ buds
- Psyllium cereal
- Oat bran
- Oats (steel cut)

Grains:
- Barley
- Bulgar
- Mung bean noodles
- Pasta
- Pulse Flours
- Quinoa
- Rice

Other:
- Peas
- Popcorn

- Sweet Potato
- Winter Squash

Fruits:
- Apple
- Apricot
- Banana (green, unripe)
- Berries
- Cantaloupe
- Grapefruit
- Honeydew Melon
- Mango
- Orange
- Peach
- Pear
- Plum
- Pomegranate
- Prunes

Beverages and Milk Alternatives:
- Almond milk
- Coconut Yogurt
- Soy Milk

Legumes:
- Baked beans
- Chickpeas
- Kidney beans
- Lentils
- Mung beans
- Romano beans
- Soybeans
- Split peas

Choose food **medium on the Glycemic Index (56 to 69)** less often.

These include:

Breads:
- Chapati
- Flaxseed bread
- Pita bread
- Pumpernickel bread
- Roti
- Rye bread
- Stone ground whole
- Wheat bread
- Whole grain wheat bread

Cereal:
- Cream of Wheat™ (regular)
- Oats (instant)
- Oats (large flake)
- Rye crisp crackers

Fruits:
- Banana (ripe, yellow)

- Oats (quick)

Grains and Starches:
- Basmati rice
- Brown rice
- Cornmeal
- Couscous
- Rice noodles
- White rice
- Wild rice

Other:
- Beets
- Corn
- French fries
- Parsnip
- Potato

- Cherries
- Cranberries
- Figs
- Grapes

- Kiwi
- Lychee
- Pineapple
- Raisins

Legumes:
- Lentil soup (ready-made)
- Split-pea soup (ready-made)

Choose food **high on the Glycemic Index (70 or more)** least often.

These include:

Bread:
- White
- Naan

Cereal:
- All-Bran Flakes™ cereal
- Corn Flakes™ cereal
- Cream of Wheat™ (instant)
- Puffed wheat cereal
- Rice Krispies™ cereal
- Special K™ cereal

Grains:
- Jasmine rice
- Millet
- Sticky rice
- White rice (instant)

Other:
- Carrots
- Potato (instant mashed)
- Pretzels
- Rice cakes
- Soda crackers

Although carbohydrates are the most important macronutrient for your body to function effectively, it's important to speak to a registered dietician, or certified nutrition professional, about the best intake for your personal needs.

88

2) Protein

The body is made up of mostly protein. It is the main structural component of muscle, brain, nerve tissue, blood, skin and hair. Protein is a transportation mechanism for vitamins, minerals, fat and oxygen. It is essential for acid-base balance, builds and repairs tissues, hormone and enzyme production and helps to sustain the energy provided by carbohydrates.

Protein is not a preferred fuel source for the body. However, the body will break down proteins for energy (as protein will yield four calories per gram) if you are starving and lacking carbohydrates and fat.

Many people who are not trained in the science of nutrition, wonder how a plant-based diet provides the body with enough protein. This is one of the main questions many vegans are asked. However, once you know the structural components of plants it is clear to see that they provide more than enough protein.

Think back to high school biology. Do you remember learning about plants, how the cells function and what they are made of? It's a very simple concept. Anything with a living cell contains amino acids, which are the building blocks of protein. So, all living food contains protein.

What about the starving kids in the world? People sometimes ask. Aren't they protein deficient? Yes, they are because they are starving. Anyone who lacks sufficient calories to sustain basic metabolic functions are protein deficient. But if you eat a well-balanced diet it is likely you will have more than enough protein to support body function, sustain and gain muscle mass.

If you have ever tried to eat a vegan diet and found your energy levels plummet, this is usually because you've not eaten enough calories, not because you are low in protein.

Think about some of the largest mammals like gorillas, elephants and the hippopotamus. They are herbivores and eat nothing but plant foods yet they are strong, powerful and seem to have more than enough protein in their diets.

The non-essential amino acids the body produces are alanine, asparagine, aspartic acid, cysteine, glutamic acid, glutamine, glycine, proline, serine and tyrosine (University of Arizona, 2003).

There are eight to 10 essential amino acids that cannot be made by the body and need to be consumed in the diet. These are arginine, histidine, isoleucine, leucine, lysine, methionine, phenylalanine, threonine, tryptophan, and valine (University of Arizona, 2003)

Protein quality is determined by assessing amino-acid composition, or its digestibility and bioavailability, which is how well the amino acid can be used by the body.

People often believe that animal protein is the only source of complete protein. However, there are many plant-based sources of complete protein, such as soy, quinoa, buckwheat and sprouts. Not only are these foods easier for the body to digest but also don't contain the saturated fat found in animal-products.

A well-rounded, whole-food, plant-based diet will allow for complete proteins to be made by eating a variety of incomplete proteins. The old belief was that a person eating a vegetarian or vegan diet needed to eat different incomplete proteins, such as grains with nuts, or legumes with dairy to make up a complete protein. But this is not true. As long as a variety of these foods are eaten in the diet, the body knows how to put them together to make the compete proteins as it needs them.

Recommended Intake

The average person requires only about 0.8 grams of protein per kilogram of body weight, endurance athletes about 1.2 grams per kilogram of body weight and strength athletes need a maximum of 1.7 grams of protein per kilogram of body weight (Potgieter, 2012). As a percentage breakdown, it's recommended that protein make up 10 to 35 percent of the total diet (The National Academies of Sciences Engineering Medicine, 2002). These numbers may vary based on individual goals.

It's easy to get enough protein in the diet. However, if you eat more protein than what you need, your body will either excrete it or store excess as fat. Excess protein, as seen in high-protein, low-carb diets often results in detrimental health risks. These diets promote the idea of fat loss through the production of ketones.

Ketones are waste products that result from the body metabolizing fat. Although fat loss is something many people desire, placing the body in a state of ketosis is dangerous because it causes an increase blood acidity levels. This acidic state may result in the wasting away of muscle tissue, inflammation, gout, high cholesterol, heart stress, liver damage, constipation, vitamin deficiency, exhaustion, bone damage, tooth decay and increase risk of cancer (Clement, 1998).

Although, protein is an essential nutrient and is required by the body to perform many vital functions, you don't need as much as some people will have you believe.

To figure out how much protein you need in grams per day, use this equation:

Protein requirements (g) = Weight in kilograms (KG) x recommended grams of protein (0.8 - 1.7g)

For example, if you weigh 150 pounds and you are an average active person, divide your weight by 2.2 to get kilograms (150/2.2 = 68.1 KG). Then, multiply this number by 0.8 to get your daily requirements of protein in grams (68.1 x 0.8 = 54.5).

Based on this equation, we can see that a person weighing 150 pounds only needs to eat 54.5 grams of protein per day. This isn't much when you consider that one cup of chickpeas has up to 39 grams of protein. That's over half of what the person in this example needs to eat per day in just one meal!

Plant-Based Sources Of Protein

When making the switch to a plant-based diet it is essential to know which foods provide a high amount of protein to ensure adequate intake. However, just eating enough calories of whole, plant-based food will often provide you with more than enough protein.

This list will provide you with an understanding of the protein content of many plant-based foods from highest to lower content.

Seitan: 31 grams per ½ cup serving

Seitan is a high-protein, low carbohydrate, low fat, plant-based meat alternative made from vital wheat gluten. It is simple to make and can be purchased in stores and restaurants as part of a healthy vegan meal plan.

Peanuts: 19 grams per ½ cup serving

Peanuts and peanut butter are not only high in protein but also make a delicious snack when paired with an apple or celery. Eating organic peanuts and peanut butter will help reduce your exposure to aflotoxin, which is a mould found on many peanuts. Spread onto a slice of whole-wheat bread and you have a complete protein meal.

Chickpeas: 19 grams per ½ cup serving

Chickpeas, also called garbanzo beans, are high in protein and fibre and support healthy digestion. This delicious, protein rich bean is the main ingredient in hummus. Spread hummus on a piece of whole-wheat bread and top with avocado, celery, salt and pepper for a protein-rich meal.

Edamame: 17 grams per ½ cup serving (cooked)

Edamame is another name for the soybean. It is a source of complete protein, high in fibre and makes a delicious appetizer. Many people are afraid of soy due to bad press. However, it's one of the richest sources of complete plant-based protein. However, genetically modified soy has been shown to cause health issues. Therefore, be sure to always consume organic and non-GMO soy products.

Tempeh: 16 grams per ½ cup serving

This plant-based food is made from fermented soybeans. It has more fibre than tofu and is a popular choice for vegetarians and vegans as it is versatile and can be used as a meat alternative.

Tofu: 8 to 15 grams per ½ cup serving

This is a classic plant-based food made from curdled soy milk. It's not as high in protein as tempeh, or edamame, but is often preferred due to its smooth texture. Tofu is versatile and can be used in sweet or savoury dishes.

Almonds: 15 grams per ½ cup serving

Almonds are not only a great source of protein they are also rich in vitamin E, magnesium and calcium. Almonds are lower in fat than some other nuts so it's best to eat them sprouted to release the nutrients. **To sprout:** soak almonds in filtered water for two to six hours. Drain the water, rinse and dry with a towel. The sprouting process allows the enzymes to come alive making it easier for the body to digest and assimilate the nutrients. Refrigerate for up to five days.

Steel-Cut Oats: 14 grams in ½ cup serving (dry)

Steel-cut oats are a good source of protein but are probably better known as a complex, fibre rich carbohydrate.

Wild Rice: 12 grams per ½ cup serving (cooked)

Wild rice is a protein-rich, complex carbohydrate source with a nutty taste and chewy texture. Black and brown rice also contain protein but not as much as wild rice.

Sunflower Sprouts: 12 grams per ½ cup serving

Sunflower sprouts are very high in protein and other essential vitamins and minerals. These sprouts are easy to grow and make a great addition to a salad or sandwich.

Cashews: 10 grams per ½ cup serving

Cashews are often used in raw, plant-based food recipes. They are rich in vitamin K and magnesium, which help build strong bones. Cashews are the perfect ingredient for making raw vegan cheesecake and other cheese-like recipes due to higher fat content.

Pumpkin Seeds: 10 grams per ½ cup serving

Pumpkin seeds are rich in magnesium, zinc and omega fatty acids. They are a perfect addition to any salad, breakfast cookie or trail mix.

Lentils: 9 grams per ½ cup serving

Lentils are high in fibre, protein and low in calories. They are often used as a meat alternative and easily transformed into delicious dips and other recipes.

Black Beans: 7.6 grams per ½ cup serving (cooked)

Black beans are packed with fibre, protein, vitamins and minerals. Black beans are versatile and can be used in many different dishes instead of ground beef.

Quinoa: 4 grams per ½ cup serving (cooked)

Quinoa is a seed but known as a pseudo grain because of its carbohydrate content. This delicious, and versatile, food is also a good source of complete plant-based protein.

Spirulina: 4 grams per tablespoon

Spirulina is an algae that is among some of the richest sources of protein and omega fats in the world. It is a nutrient dense food that is easily added to smoothies as a powder or taken in pill form.

Potatoes: 4 grams in one medium white potato

Potatoes are often thought of as being a food that is "bad" or low in nutrients but they are a good source of protein and are high in potassium. Enjoy them roasted, mashed or scalloped.

Chia Seeds: 3 grams per tablespoon

Chia seeds are rich in protein and omega fatty acids, which signals your body to burn fat rather than storing it. You can eat these seeds raw, or soak them in plant-based milk to make a delicious pudding.

Spinach: 3 grams per ½ cup serving (cooked)

Although 3 grams of protein doesn't seem like much the protein in greens is very bioavailable. Popeye had it right. It does a body good!

Corn: 2.5 grams per ½ cup serving

Corn is often thought of as a useless starch but if you pair it with other veggies and legumes it helps round out a well-balanced complete protein-based meal. For the healthiest option choose non-GMO and organic corn.

Avocado: 2 grams per ½ avocado

Avocados are a fatty fruit that contain a little protein. This food is the perfect addition to a sandwich, topping for a salad, blended for salad dressing or mashed to make **guacamole** (see recipe on page 187).

Broccoli: 2 grams per ½-cup serving (cooked)

This delicious veggie is very high in fibre and contains some protein. Eat it raw by itself or in salads or steamed.

Brussels Sprouts: 2 grams per ½-cup serving

These veggies are often given a bad rap for not having the best taste. When lightly steamed or stir-fried and topped with a delicious sauce they are a healthy delight high in potassium and vitamin k.

3) Fat

Fat provides the body with the most energy of all the macronutrients and is an important macronutrient, an essential part of a healthy, well-balanced diet. At nine calories per gram, it's best to consume fat in moderation if weight loss is a goal.

Critical functions in the body such as brain function, organ insulation, cell structure, nerve transmission, vitamin absorption and hormone production depend on fat.

Recommended Intake

Research shows that an individual may require about 0.2 to 0.4 grams of fat per pound of body weight. Total percentage of fat in the diet should be less than 30 percent. This amount will vary based on your personal health and fitness goals. For best health, less than 10 percent of the dietary fat should come from saturated fat and hydrogenated, or trans fats, which should be avoided all together (American Heart Association, 2015).

Saturated Fatty Acids (Saturated Fat)

The most well-known saturated fats come from animal products. The problem with animal fat is that it's also been shown to increase LDL (the bad) cholesterol and increase risk of atherosclerosis (clogging of the arteries) and heart disease (American Heart Association, 2015).

When cooked at high temperatures, animal fat has been shown to form chemicals that may be carcinogenic. That is, these harmful chemicals cause changes in DNA and may in crease the risk of cancer (National Cancer Institute, 2017).

The healthiest kind of saturated fat comes from coconuts as raw coconut meat, coconut butter or coconut oil. The difference between the saturated fat in animal products and that of a coconut is the chemical structure.

According to Dr. Mercola (2016), coconut oil is made up of about two-thirds medium-chain fatty acids versus long-chain fatty acids found in saturated fat from animal sources.

Coconut oil is found to be healthy because 50 percent of the fat content is lauric acid. The body breaks down lauric acid into monolaurin and then uses this compound to destroy viruses such as HIV, herpes, measles and influenza.

Coconut oil also:

- supports the healthy function of the immune, cardiovascular, nervous and endocrine systems.
- promotes weight loss and healthy metabolism
- is a sources of energy for the body
- promotes beautiful skin and healthy gums.

If you must cook with oil, coconut oil is one of the best oils to choose. It's minimally refined and has a high heat tolerance and won't break down into a hydrogenated fat as easily as other oils.

Hydrogenated (Trans) Fat

Trans fat is found to occur naturally in meat and dairy and often used to help preserve packaged foods such as:

- commercial baked goods like cookies, doughnuts, muffins, cakes, pizza dough and vegetable shortening
- snack foods such as crackers, microwave popcorn, chips and candy bars
- fried foods like french fries, fried chicken, chicken nuggets, breaded fish

Trans-fatty acid is toxic to the body and has also been shown to raise LDL (bad) cholesterol and increase risk of disease (Greger, 2019). For optimal health, it's best to refrain from eating food that contains trans fat.

Unsaturated Fat

Eating foods that contain unsaturated fat, in moderation, is advisable and supports a healthy heart and body function.

Unsaturated fats are categorized into:

- **Monounsaturated fats.** This type of fat will help increase HDL (the good) cholesterol (Greger, 2019). Foods rich in monounsaturated fat include olives, peanuts, sesame oil, avocados, cacao beans, almonds, pecans, cashews, macadamia nuts and hazelnuts.

- **Polyunsaturated fats.** This type of fat has been shown by the American Heart Association (2015) to be beneficial for the heart when eaten in moderation and used to replace saturated fat in the diet. These fats are most dominant in walnuts, sunflower, sesame, pumpkin seeds, flaxseed, hemp and tofu.

Essential Fatty Acids

Essential fatty acids include omega 3, 5, 6, 7, and 9. Omegas are unsaturated fats that need to be consumed in the diet and support a variety of health body functions (Robertson, 2017).

Omega-3 Fatty Acids

Omega-3s are polyunsaturated fats and must be consumed in the diet. Unfortunately, the typical western diet does not usually contain enough omega-3s and a deficiency may contribute to chronic diseases such as obesity, diabetes and heart disease (Robertson, 2017).

There are many types of omega-3 fats but the most common are:

- **ALA** (Alpha-Linolenic Acid) – found in a variety of plant-foods and needs to be converted into EPA or DHA before it can be used by the body.

- **EPA** (Eicosapentaenoic Acid) – Plant-based source is algae.

- **DHA** (Docosahexaenoic Acid) – Plant-based source is algae.

Health benefits of omega-3 fats include:

- Helps to reduce inflammation
- Shown to help lower risk of chronic diseases such as heart disease, cancer, and arthritis
- Highly concentrated in the brain and appear to be important for cognitive (brain memory and performance) and behavioural function
- Helps in weight management
- Prevents dementia
- Promote bone health
- Reduce asthma symptoms

Foods high in omega-3 fat include:

- Chia seeds
- Brussels sprouts
- Algae
- Hemp seed
- Walnuts
- Flaxseed

Omega-6 Fatty Acids

Omega-6s are polyunsaturated fatty acids that must be consumed in the diet. The typical western diet usually has more than enough of this type of fat as it is most often found in processed foods.

Consuming whole food rich in omega-6s promote good health but too much of this fat from processed food can promote inflammation and be detrimental to health (Robertson, 2017).

Health benefits of omega-6 fatty acids includes:

- Provides energy to the body
- Supports brain health and function
- Stimulates hair and skin growth
- Maintains good bone health
- Helps regulate metabolism
- Supports reproductive health
- Helps reduce nerve pain
- Reduces inflammation

Foods high in omega-6 fats include:

- Flaxseed
- Hemp seed
- Grapeseed oil
- Pumpkin seeds
- Sunflower seeds
- Pine nuts
- Pistachios
- Açai

Omega-9 Fatty Acids

Omega-9s are monounsaturated fats that can be produced by the body and are found in cellular tissue (Robertson, 2017).
Health benefits of omega-9 fats include:

- Support metabolic health
- Reduce LDL (the bad) cholesterol
- Improve insulin sensitivity
- Help to decrease inflammation

Foods high in omega-9 fats include:

- Olive oil
- Cashew nuts
- Almonds
- Avocado
- Peanut
- Walnuts

Omega-7 Fatty Acids

Omega-7s are newly recognized monounsaturated fats. The most common omega-7 fatty acid is palmitoleic acid.

Heath benefits of omega-7 fats include:

- Reduced inflammation
- Reduces LDL cholesterol and triglyceride levels
- Lowers insulin levels
- Improves liver function

- Promotes weight loss
- Linked to improved bowel regularity
- Rejuvenation of skin – as it is said to nourish and sustain healthy cells in the digestive tract and skin.

Foods high in omega-7 fats include:

- Olive oil
- Macadamia oil
- Sea buckthorn oil

Plant-Based Omega Versus Fish Oil: Which Is Best?

Many people eat fish and take fish supplements as a source of omega fatty acids. However, fish don't make omegas in their bodies. They must eat it just like we do. Fish eat plants, such as algae, to get omegas. So why do we eat fish to get omegas? It makes more sense and is more effective to go straight to the source. Plants.

Experts like Dr. Michael Greger (2018) state that many studies have shown that taking fish products as omega supplements may result in adverse health effects. This is likely due to the environmental contaminants, such as methyl mercury, found in certain fish. These contaminants, and their detrimental health effects, diminish any benefits of taking fish oil as a source of omega fatty acid.

Plant-based sources of omegas do not contain mercury and radiation contaminants and offer the same health benefits.

In his book Killer Fish (2014), Dr. Brian Clement, provides many reasons why humans should not eat fish and other aquatic life.

These reasons include:

- Fish meat contains saturated fat.

- Fish and other seafood are riddled with industrial waste products, environmental contaminants like mercury and radiation, pharmaceutical drugs, parasites and amoebas.

- The consumption of fish in the diet has been shown to increase the chances of heart disease, strokes, neurological deficits, cancer, auto-immune and endocrine disorders.

- Farm-raised fish have significantly higher levels of toxins than fish found in nature.

After looking at the research about the risks of consuming fish and fish products, especially now with factory farming and environmental pollutants, like any other meat, fish is not a health food and should be avoided.

107

Saturated vs. Unsaturated Fat Comparison Chart

	Saturated Fat	Unsaturated Fat
Type of bonds	Single bond	At least one double bond
Recommended consumption	No more than 10% of total calories per day	No more that 30% of total calories per day (this may vary depending on individual needs and requirements
Health effects	Too much consumption has shown to increase atherosclerosis and heart disease	High in antioxidants and promote healthy cholesterol
Cholesterol	Increase Low Density Lipoproteins (LDL or bad cholesterol)	Increase High Density Lipoprotein (HDL or good cholesterol)
Commonly found in	Butter, whole milk, meat, peanut butter, margarine, cheese, fried foods, frozen dinners, and vegetable oil. Coconut oil is a saturated fat but has a different chemical structure than animal fat. It has been shown to promote better health	Avocado, hemp, chia, flax and other seeds, sunflower and soybean oil, which should only be consumed if non-GMO & organic.
Melting point	High	Low
Physical state at room temperature	Solid	Liquid
Rancidity	Low	High

** Chart developed from a variety of resources

What Are Micronutrients?

Micronutrients include vitamins, minerals, antioxidants and phytochemicals. These are the non-calorie nutrients that enable the body to produce enzymes, hormones and other functions essential for proper growth, development and health.

When we consume enough micronutrients from real whole food we have optimal health and function. However, when the diet lacks these essential nutrients the consequences can be severe and result in debilitating chronic disease and even death.

The three categories of micronutrients and their components include:

1) Vitamins

Vitamins are an organic material, which means they can break down and easily be destroyed. For the most part, vitamins must be consumed in the diet daily.

Not one food contains all the essential vitamins we need for optimal health, which is why it is important to eat a well-balanced diet rich in whole, real food. Some foods, such as cereals and breads, are now fortified with vitamins to help prevent deficiency resulting from a poor diet.

Vitamins are divided into two categories: water and fat soluble vitamins.

Water Soluble Vitamins

Water-soluble vitamins require water to be transported around the body. It's unlikely to have an overdose of these vitamins, as any excess will be excreted in the urine.

Water-soluble vitamins:

- **Thiamin (vitamin B1)** helps the body release energy from carbohydrates during metabolism, supports nerve function and the growth and tone of muscle tissue (American Council on Exercise, 2014). Plant-based sources of vitamin B1 include fortified cereals, rice, pasta and whole grains.

- **Riboflavin (vitamin B2)** helps the body release energy from protein, fat and carbohydrates during metabolism. It is also considered an antioxidant and helps to prevent oxidation, or destruction, of cellular tissue (American Council on Exercise, 2014). Plant-based sources of vitamin B2 include whole grains and dark leafy vegetables.

- **Niacin (vitamin B3)** supports the metabolism of carbohydrate, fat and protein (American Council on Exercise, 2014). Plant-based sources of vitamin B3 include enriched cereals, peanuts and potatoes.

- **Pantothenic acid (vitamin B5)** is present in all plant and animal tissue and is essential for metabolism of fat, protein and carbohydrates (American Council on Exercise, 2014). Plant-based sources of this vitamin include whole grains, legumes, vegetables and fruit.

- **Pyridoxine (vitamin B6)** helps support protein and carbohydrate metabolism, production of red blood cells, supports immune function and helps build body tissue (American Council on Exercise, 2014). Plant-based sources of vitamin B6 include bananas, prunes, beans, whole grains and avocados.

- **Folate (vitamin B9)** helps with the production of DNA, formation of red and white blood cells and neurotransmitters and metabolism of amino acids (American Council on Exercise, 2014). Plant-based sources of vitamin B9 include green leafy vegetables, peas, beans and lentils.

- **Cobalamin (vitamin B12)** is required for the normal development and cellular function in the digestive tract, bone marrow and nervous tissue as well as metabolism of protein and fat (American Council on Exercise, 2014). Plant-based sources of vitamin B12 include fermented foods such as sauerkraut, kimchi and kombucha.

- **Biotin (vitamin B7)** plays an important role in the metabolic functions of pantothenic acid, folic acid, vitamin B12 and metabolism of proteins, fats and carbohydrates (American Council on Exercise, 2014). Vitamin B7 can be produced by healthy intestinal flora (bacteria) but can also be found in plant-based food such as cereal or grain products, brewers and nutritional yeast and legumes.

- **Ascorbic Acid (vitamin C)** is a powerful antioxidant and is essential for the structure of bones, cartilage, muscle and blood vessels, maintaining the health of capillaries, teeth, gums and aids in the absorption of iron (American Council on Exercise, 2014). Plant-based sources of vitamin C include citrus fruits, berries and vegetables.

Fat-Soluble Vitamins

Fat-soluble vitamins require fat for transportation around the body. However, be sure not to consume too much of these vitamins. Any excess that has not been excreted will be stored in the liver, or fat tissue, until needed. This can increase risk of overdose and toxicity.

It is possible to consume all the required fat-soluble vitamins on a vegan diet. All you need to do is eat a well-balanced diet rich in a variety of whole food.

112

Fat-soluble vitamins:

- **Vitamin A** contains beta-carotene, which is important for vision, growth of bones and teeth and the formation and maintenance of skin, hair and mucus membranes (American Council on Exercise, 2014). Plant-based sources of vitamin A include yellow and orange fruits and vegetables, green leafy vegetables and fortified oatmeal.

- **Vitamin D** is essential for calcium and phosphorous absorption, to maintain homeostasis, aids in bone and tooth formation and helps maintain heart and nervous system function (American Council on Exercise, 2014). Small amounts of sun exposure help the body produce this vitamin but it can also be obtained from supplements and fortified foods.

- **Vitamin E,** also known as alpha-tocopherol, is a powerful antioxidant and plays a fundamental role in protecting blood cells, body tissue and essential fatty acids from destruction in the body (American Council on Exercise, 2014). Plant-based sources of vitamin E include fortified cereal, nuts, wheat germ, vegetable oils and green leafy vegetables.

- **Vitamin K** is important for blood clotting and maintenance of strong bones (American Council on Exercise, 2014). It is produced by bacteria in the colon but can also be found in green leafy vegetables, fruit and grain products.

2) Minerals

Minerals are critical for human life and are found in the body as well as in food. Minerals are typically categorized as macro-minerals (major elements) and micro-minerals (trace elements).

Macro-minerals:

- **Calcium** is the most abundant mineral in the human body and helps to mineralize bones and teeth, muscle contraction (including the heart), blood clotting, control of blood pressure and supports immunity (American Council on Exercise, 2014). Plant-based sources of calcium include green leafy vegetables, legumes, nuts and the cacao bean.

- **Phosphorous** plays a role in bone and teeth health, helps the kidneys filter waste and is important for the use of protein, fat and carbohydrates (American Council on Exercise, 2014). The main plant-based food sources of phosphorous include grains.

- **Magnesium** is present in bone, muscle, soft tissue and body fluids and is important for bone mineralization, protein production,

114

muscle contraction, nerve conduction, enzyme function and healthy teeth (American Council on Exercise, 2014). Plant-based sources of magnesium include nuts, cacao bean, green vegetables and whole grains.

- **Sulfur** is important for bonding proteins and enzyme and other body functions (American Council on Exercise, 2014). Plant-based sources of sulfur include beans, broccoli, cauliflower, Brussels sprouts, mustard greens, bok choy, onions, garlic, celery, fennel and asparagus.

- **Sodium** is one of three electrolytes in the body and is important for normal cellular function, water balance and distribution and acid-base balance (American Council on Exercise, 2014). Plant-based sources of sodium include artichokes, celery, beets, turnips, chard, sweet potatoes and spinach.

- **Chloride** is one of three electrolytes in the body and is important for normal cellular function, water balance and distribution and acid-base balance (American Council on Exercise, 2014). Plant-based sources of chloride include sea salt, tomatoes, leafy greens, seaweed, olives and rye.

- **Potassium** is one of three electrolytes in the body and is important for normal cellular function, water balance and distribution and acid-base balance (American Council on Exercise, 2014). Plant-based sources of potassium include squash, potatoes, beans, oranges, broccoli, bananas, lentils, raisins and pistachios.

Micro-minerals:

- **Iron** is responsible for hemoglobin formation, improves blood quality and helps the body resist stress and disease (American Council on Exercise, 2014). Plant-based sources of iron include legumes, grains, nuts, seeds, dark leafy greens, prunes and blackstrap molasses.

- **Iodine** is a mineral stored in the thyroid gland and is responsible for normal growth and metabolism (American Council on Exercise, 2014). Plant-based sources of iodine include sea vegetables, potatoes, prunes, bananas, corn, cranberries, green beans and strawberries.

- **Selenium** is a powerful antioxidant and protects the body against oxidative damage from radiation, pollution and normal metabolic processing (American Council on Exercise, 2014). Plant-based sources of selenium include grains, nuts, seeds, baked beans, mushrooms, oatmeal, spinach, lentils and bananas.

- **Zinc** stimulates the activity of enzymes, supports a healthy immune system, assists with wound healing, strengthens the taste and smell senses,

116

supports normal growth and development and helps with DNA synthesis (American Council on Exercise, 2014). Plant-based sources of zinc include whole grains, tofu, lentils, hemp seeds, oatmeal, rice, seeds, beans, quinoa, mushrooms and avocados.

3) Antioxidants & Phytochemicals

Vitamins and minerals act like powerful antioxidants. However, there are many more antioxidants and phytochemicals found in fresh, whole food that support good health.

Antioxidants have been proven to prevent and repair cellular tissue damage. This destruction of cellular tissue is caused by free radicals and is the result of excessive inflammation and toxic exposure. A poor diet high in processed foods, sugar and saturated fats and low in whole foods rich in vitamins and minerals, smoking, as well as environmental pollutants like radiation increases the risk of damage caused by free radicals.

Think of oxidative stress like this. If you cut an apple in half and leave it on the counter it will start to turn brown. This is the result of cellular tissue breakdown from oxidative stress.

If you place lemon juice on the cut apple, you will notice that the it will not brown as quickly. The antioxidants in the lemon help protect the cellular tissue of the apple.

117

The same is true in the body. When we eat enough antioxidants, the body has the protection it needs to fight off free radicals. The more antioxidants the more protection the body has from cellular damage, disease and the aging process (Haytowitz & Bhagwat, 2010).

Some of the benefits of consuming antioxidant foods include (Axe, 2018):

- Reduced signs of aging and longer life span
- Reduced risk of cancer, heart disease, stroke, vision and cognitive problems
- Detoxification
- Glowing and younger looking skin

Currently, there is no recommended daily allowance (RDA) value set for antioxidants. The level of antioxidants is measured by what's called an ORAC Scale (oxygen radical absorption capacity), which tests the power of a plant to absorb and eliminate free radicals (Haytowitz & Bhagwat, 2010).

Some of the top 10 foods high in antioxidants (measurements based on 100 grams of each item) include (Axe, 2018):

1) Goji berries – 25,000 ORAC Score

2) Wild blueberries – 14,000 ORAC Score

3) Dark chocolate – 21,000 ORAC Score

4) Pecans – 17,000 ORAC Score

5) Elderberries – 14,000 ORAC Score

6) Artichoke – 9,400 ORAC Score

7) Kidney beans – 8,400 ORAC Score

8) Cranberries – 9,500 ORAC Score

9) Blackberries – 2,036 ORAC Score

10) Cilantro - 5,100 ORAC Score

Phytochemicals are nutrients in plants not necessarily required for normal functioning but improve health and reduce risk of disease.

For example, there are over 10,000 phytochemicals in one apple alone! It is no wonder the old saying, "an apple a day keeps the doctor away," is so true.

When you eat a variety of whole foods, which all have tens of thousands of phytochemicals, including vitamins, minerals and antioxidants, you will have more energy, healthier teeth, hair, nails and skin, reduced weight and a decreased risk for getting a chronic disease.

How To Get Enough Micronutrients In Your Diet

The solution to a healthy body is really not that hard. It just takes preparation and adjusting the taste buds

119

to prefer whole foods instead of processed foods high in sugar, fat and salt.

Here are some simple ways to boost your nutrition intake and your overall health:

1) Follow The New Canada Food Guide System

The new Canada Food Guide (Government of Canada, 2019) is an easy visual of what to have on your plate. Essentially the suggestion is to have half of your plate vegetables and fruit, with more being vegetables, a quarter of your plate protein and a quarter of your plate whole grains and other healthy, complex carbohydrates. Replacing drinks such as juices, pop and milk with water will also help cut down on empty calories and sugar and help the body stay better hydrated.

2) Plan Ahead

Take time to plan your meals, purchase ingredients and make the food you want to eat for a few days. This will save you time and the temptation to make unhealthy choices.

A good way to start this process is to decide what you'd like to make for the week. Buy most of the ingredients that day. Cut up everything you will eat raw and cook what needs to be cooked. Store this food in sealed containers in the fridge or freezer until you're ready to eat.

Having your food ready in grab-and-go containers or bags will save time and allow you to enjoy the healthy food you set out to eat.

3) Get Creative

One of the biggest mistakes I see people make with their diet is eating the same thing each day. Although it is a simple way to keep track of calories, it's easy to fall off your healthy eating plan because of boredom and intense cravings for other foods. Therefore, find some delicious new recipes, like the ones in this book, you want to try and get creative with your meals. Experts suggest that eating a variety of plant-foods is good for the gut and will produce the best results for you health.

4) Drink Smoothies

Smoothies are an easy way to get a variety of fruits and veggies and other nutrients in your diet because you can put all sorts of delicious ingredients into the blender and drink it, rather than just eat all that food.

Some of my favourite smoothies, like the ones found in the recipe section of this book (page 175) include spinach, kale, banana, frozen fruit, hemp, chia and flax seeds, coconut milk and sometimes a scoop of protein powder.

5) Supplements

It's often hard to get enough nutrients from food

because the food quality is poor from suboptimal growing conditions or travel time, from the lack of variety or ability to eat whole food. Therefore, supplementation, either through fortification of foods or dietary supplements is necessary.

Many supplements, such as multivitamins and many protein supplements on the market have been proven to cause more harm than good. Unfortunately, many supplements are not regulated, tested or approved by Health Canada and often contain harmful ingredients not listed on the label.

We're lucky to live in a day and age where supplementation is an option. However, it's extremely important to know the supplements you are taking. Take time to research each supplement, understand the ingredients and where they have been sourced and learn a little about the company who makes them. Find out if they are a company that conducts business in an ethical manner and care about using healthy ingredients.

Chapter 7:
Essential Tools For Your Kitchen

I'm sure you will agree that spending time in the kitchen is much more fun when you have the right tools. Proper kitchen tools will make life easier and more enjoyable so you can create the best-tasting meals with ease.

Many years ago I took a raw-vegan chef certification course because I was obsessed with learning how to make the most delicious, yet healthy, meals while I was writing my first cookbook.

However, as I was cutting up numerous veggies and trying to prepare these dishes I was frustrated with my cheap, dull knives, my food processor that burned out on me every second use and my blender that hardly broke food down.

I researched a variety of knives, blenders, food processors, juicers and other tools that are must-haves in the kitchen and decided it was time to up my game and invest in some decent kitchen equipment and tools.

To make spending time in the kitchen creating new delicious recipes here is a collection of some of the essential tools you will want to have in your kitchen.

1) A high-quality knife set

Using a good quality knife when it comes to cutting, peeling and chopping, is life-changing. When I got my first really good set of knives all I wanted to do was chop veggies. Suddenly, this was a fun task that so many people hate doing.

Although high-quality knives require some initial investment they are worth every penny and usually come with an excellent guarantee.

You don't need to start with a full set, just choose one or two knives you think you would use the most and start there.

The knives to have in your collection include:

- **Chef's knife** - This multi-purpose knife is designed for many different needs including mincing, slicing, and chopping vegetables.

- **Santoku knife** – This general, all-purpose knife is most often used for chopping, dicing and mincing. It is designed to provide a comfortable and well-balanced grip.

- **Paring knife** – This small knife is perfect for peeling and chopping fruits and vegetables.

124

It's often one of the most used knives in the kitchen, next to the chef's knife.

- **Bread knife** – This serrated knife is great for cutting through crusty bread and vegetables like tomatoes.

2) High-speed blender

If you don't have a Vitamix™ you are missing out. My friends and clients have called me the smoothie master because every time I do a smoothie-making party, people are delighted by how smooth and tasty my smoothies are.

As much as I want to take all the credit, I can't. Yes, I know how to add the perfect ratio of ingredients into the blender but place these same ingredients in a regular blender and it just wouldn't be the same.

My preferred choice and recommended blender is by far the Vitamix™. This blender, and any other decent blender, is a considerable investment but it's worth it!

There are many things you can do with a good high-speed blender. You can make smoothies, soups, dressings and so much more and it will come with a collection of recipes to help get you started.

3) High-quality food processor

You may not think you need a food processor, especially one that costs a few hundred dollars, but when you get it you will wonder what you ever did without it.

Sure you can work with a cheap, low quality food processor. However, if you use it a lot you will likely burn out the motor.

Imagine this. You are in the creative process and the perfect dish is coming together nicely. You have all the ingredients in your food processor, you press the button, it starts going and then suddenly it stops. What are you going to do? You have company coming over and you want to make the perfect dinner. So, you rush out to the store and end up buying one of the top models in the store to ensure this never happens again.

This may not have happened to you but it has happened to me.

When I started using a new, high-quality food processor it was much better that I vowed to inspire others to invest in a good one so they didn't have to experience what I went through.

My favourite food processor right now is the Cuisinart™. When I did my research it looks like the Kitchen Aid™ is close in quality and likely also a great choice.

4) Mandolin slicer

I have to admit, although I do use my mandolin slicer

a lot, I still like to cut my veggies using my good knives. However, if you are cutting up large amounts of veggies, and you want them cut perfectly or in a special way such as julienne, french fries or a flat cut, the mandolin slicer is the best tool to have on hand.

Just a word of caution. Be sure to use the hand guard because if you don't, you may slice off a finger, or at least a nail.

5) Juicer

I started my plant-based journey by drinking fruit and vegetable juice every day. There is nothing like a freshly made green juice. It is very refreshing, hydrating and nourishing.

Juicers range from about $100 to $3000. I personally don't think it's necessary to spend thousands of dollars on a juicer when a less expensive one will do just fine but it does depend on what you want to juice.

Two types of juicers exist, the centrifugal juicer and the slow juicer.

Centrifugal juice extractors are the most common type of home juicer. A fast-spinning blade spins against a mesh filter using centrifugal force to pull the juice from the flesh of the fruits or vegetables.

127

The problem with this type of juicer is the speed at which the juice is extracted destroys some of the enzymes and the heat may oxidize the nutrients in the fruits and vegetables.

The benefit of this juicer is that it is more affordable than the cold press, or slow juicer.

If you want to juice root veggies and fruits a centrifugal juicer, like a Breville™, will work well.

The cold press, masticating juicer or slow juicer, extracts the juice by crushing and pressing the fruit and vegetables to yield the most juice. Because no heat is produced during the juicing process all enzymes and nutrients stay intact.

This type of juicer, like a Hurom™ or Omega™, is excellent for juicing dark leafy greens, making fresh nut milks and is quieter than a centrifugal juicer.

Although this is the better juicer it is a significant investment as it is more expensive.

For wheat grass, I suggest a slow juicer or a wheat-grass specific juicer specially designed to only juice wheatgrass for best results.

6) Dehydrator

A dehydrator is a tool you can use to dry out food to keep it raw. To keep food raw it must be cooked at temperatures lower than 118°F.

Until I became a raw-vegan chef I had no idea what kinds of raw foods I could make in the dehydrator. Snacks like kale chips, raw crackers, dried fruit and granola taste much better when they've been dehydrated as opposed to cooked in the oven as the nutrients have been left in tact.

My favourite dehydrator is the Excalibur™. It costs about $400, depending on the size you get, but it's well worth the money!

7) Spiralizer

A spiralizer is a fun tool to have in the kitchen. This tool will have you making fancy raw zucchini dishes and topping salads like a professional chef with spiralled carrots and beets.

There are many different types of spiralizers. Some can get pretty pricey but you can get basic ones at an affordable price.

8) Glass jars

I am a big fan of mason jars or glass jars in general. I use them for many things. The large mason jars, which are about one litre, are perfect for sprouting seeds such as sunflower, buckwheat and pea shoots.

Keep flour, sugar, spices and other ingredients that usually come in a bag in these jars so your cupboards look tidy and clean. You may also use them to store your to-go meals!

9) Cutting boards

Since you will have your beautiful new set of knives a nice cutting board will be essential to preserve the life of your knives.

I prefer wood cutting boards, as they are easier on the knives. Glass ones, although really easy to clean and look nice, will dull your knives.

A nice quality wood cutting board can be an investment but like any other kitchen tool it's worth it.

10) Pots and pans

Any chef will tell you that having a nice set of pots and pans is well worth the investment.

I would suggest finding a high-quality set you really like and purchase one-piece-at-a-time until you have the entire set. Unless you decide to just buy the whole thing up front. That's always a great option too!

Some key pieces to start with include:

- **Large pot -** A large pot is good for making soups, boiling potatoes, cooking pasta and popping popcorn.

- **Small pot -** A small pot is good for heating up leftovers, making oatmeal and other small dishes.

130

- **Steamer set** - A steamer set, or even a removable steamer basket, is good for steaming veggies and edamame beans.

- **Large skillet** - A large skillet is good for sautéing vegetables and making stir-fry.

- **Small skillet** - A small skillet is good for heating leftovers or making small batches of sautéed vegetables.

11) Bake ware

Once you go meatless you will likely be excited to make all your favourite desserts plant-based style.

This is why you will want to have some nice bake ware pieces in your kitchen.

Some of the basics you will want to have handy include:

- **Mixing bowls** – Mixing bowls are good all-purpose bowls and are good for mixing muffins, cakes, cookie batter or tossing and serving salad.

- **Baking pans** (one large and two small) – Baking pans are good for baking cakes, cooking plant-based meat alternatives or potatoes and heating leftovers.

- **Cookie sheet** – A cookie sheet is good for baking cookies.

- **Muffin tin** – A muffin tin is essential for baking muffins and to use for dishes like raw cashew cheesecake.

- **Spring-form pan** – A spring form pan is good for baking cakes or making raw vegan cheesecakes.

12) Measuring tools

A good set of measuring cups and spoons is a lifesaver when you are making the perfect dish.

Some essential measuring tools include:

- **Measuring cups** - Measuring cups are useful for measuring liquid, such as plant-based milk and vegetable broth, or dry ingredients, like flour and sugar, for a variety of dishes.

- **Measuring spoons** – Measuring spoons are also useful for liquid, such as vanilla extract, or dry ingredients, like spices, for a variety of dishes.

13) Spatulas, wooden spoons and flippers

Spatulas, wooden spoons and flippers are essential must-have tools for your kitchen. Without them you won't be able to stir, mix or flip your delicious food.

132

I know for many years I used old spatulas, spoons and flippers that I had been handed down from my mom. However, when I invested in a whole new set it was an elevated cooking experience.

There is something special about having all your favourite tools ready and waiting to be used. When you pick them up you feel like you really belong in the kitchen.

It's these simple pleasures that will keep you coming back to the kitchen and preparing delicious, healthy, whole food meals.

14) Storage containers

A big part of making fresh meals and eating at home is the leftovers! Some dishes taste better the next day after all the spices and flavours have had time to soak in.

This is why you will need a good set of storage containers. Small ones are perfect for storing chopped veggies. Medium containers are nice for packing lunches. Large containers are great for storing baked goods or large batches of rice to use over the course of a few days.

Unless you can find a high-quality plastic that is BPA-free, glass storage containers are the best.

15) Love

I know, love isn't really a tool. However; I believe it's an essential part of the cooking process.

Many years ago when I was dealing with an eating disorder, I was advised to start cooking. The premise was to learn to love the food I was preparing, understand as much as I could about different ingredients and prepare the food with love while enjoying the process. The purpose of this exercise was to learn to love the food I was putting in my body rather than hate it.

The energy of love brings a light energy to the food that you can actually taste. And when you make food for the people you love, including yourself, you are not only feeding them you are also feeding your soul.

You're all set! Now that you have all the essential tools you need for your vegan kitchen you are ready to get cooking!

Chapter 8:
Suggested Ingredients

It can be frustrating to find the perfect recipe only to discover you don't have any of the ingredients. That's why in this chapter, you will learn about a few ingredients to have on hand so you're ready to make a variety of healthy and delicious meals at home rather than be tempted to eat out.

Where To Start

Have you ever opened the fridge and stared blankly into the large box thinking, "there's nothing in here to eat." Then you close the door and reach for a bag of crackers or chips, which only leaves you feeling completely unfulfilled and still hungry.

That's exactly how I used to feel before becoming vegan. Now, when I look in the fridge, as long as I have a few key ingredients, there is always something that can be pulled together to make a delicious and healthy meal.

Once you get your kitchen stocked with a variety of key ingredients your thought will change from, "I have nothing to eat," to, "oh my goodness, there's so much here where do I even begin? What do I want to eat? What recipes do I get to make tonight?" Suddenly, cooking will become a fun and exciting adventure.

Suggested Ingredients For Your Vegan Kitchen

Eating a whole food plant-based diet to support your calorie and nutrient needs, so you can stay active and healthy, doesn't have to be hard. With a few simple ingredients you can prepare quick, simple meals or experiment with fancier recipes for a gourmet meal that will impress any guest.

Here are a few essential ingredients that are must-haves for your kitchen:

Fresh & Frozen Produce

A healthy plant-based kitchen will always be stocked full of a variety of fresh produce. It gets easy, when first going meatless, to eat a lot of processed foods because there are so many options on the market today. However, just because you choose to live an animal-free diet doesn't mean you should neglect your health.

I believe fresh and frozen produce is essential because sometimes, in the winter months, frozen produce is a better option. It is allowed to fully ripen

136

and then is flash frozen at peak nutritional value. Frozen is also convenient and lasts longer than fresh produce.

Some essential fresh and frozen foods to have on-hand at all times include:

Spinach

Spinach is an essential leafy green. It is high in vitamins and minerals, especially calcium and it's a good source of protein. Spinach is an excellent addition to smoothies.

Kale

Kale is a hearty and healthy leafy green. Kale salads and kale chips are a nice way to eat this vegetable.

Romaine and other lettuce

Romaine, and other lettuce varieties make a nice base for any salad, topping for a sandwich or as a substitute to a bun.

Fresh parsley

Parsley is a fresh addition to salads and is known to be a natural breath freshener. Feed this to your dog daily to get rid of doggy breath.

137

Fresh basil

Basil is most often known for its use in Italian cuisine. This fresh herb, like all other herbs, contains many antioxidants and is known for its anti-inflammatory properties. If you don't have fresh basil but looking to add some flavour to a dressing or other dish you may choose to use a basil essential oil.

Fresh cilantro

Cilantro has a very distinct flavour and is one that people either love or hate. Cilantro is a great addition to salads, guacamole and Mexican cuisine. Like basil, if you don't have fresh cilantro but want to add a little flavour to your dish you may choose to use a cilantro essential oil.

Carrots

Carrots are rich in vitamin A, which supports good eyesight. They also contain a variety of antioxidants and other nutrients.

Beets

Beets, due to their rich red colour, are known to be good for the heart and blood. Beets are delicious raw in salads, smoothies and roasted in the oven with other root vegetables.

138

Cucumbers

Cucumbers make a nice light snack and as a flavour addition to water. This crunchy veggie is high in water content, natural sodium and other nutrients. Eating cucumbers may lead to many potential health benefits, including weight loss, balanced hydration, digestive regularity and lower blood sugar levels.

Frozen mixed veggies

Having a bag of frozen mixed veggies on hand is a great way to have a quick meal. You can add them to a stir-fry, shepherd's pie or simply steam the veggies. Add a little seasoning and enjoy a nice, light lunch.

Edamame

These whole soybeans are packed with complete protein and make a nice snack when looking for a quick meal.

Potatoes

Potatoes, especially sweet potatoes, are rich in a variety of vitamins and minerals and energy-giving carbohydrates. Potatoes are very versatile and can be simply roasted, baked, mashed or scalloped.

Lemons

Lemons are powerful antioxidants. Drink lemon water on an empty stomach and this will help cleanse the digestive tract. Lemon is also a great addition to any salad dressing or roasted potato dish.

Variety of fresh fruit such as bananas, apples, pears.

It is important, for a healthy kitchen to be stocked with a variety of fresh seasonal fruit. Fruit is an essential source of a variety of nutrients and make a nice sweet, yet healthy, snack.

Frozen fruit such as mangoes, blueberries and mixed berries.

Frozen fruit is nice to have in the freezer at all times as frozen fruit makes the best smoothies. You can also add frozen fruit to muffins, pancakes and other desserts.

Nuts & Seeds

Having a variety of nuts and seeds on hand will provide you with a quick, on-the-go healthy snack. Nuts and seeds are often used in recipes such as raw desserts and pâté.

Some of the best nuts and seeds to have on hand include:

Hemp seeds

Hemp seeds are high in protein and omega fatty acids. They can be sprinkled on salads, oatmeal or

140

added to smoothies.

Chia seeds

Chia seeds are high in protein and omega fatty acids. They can be sprinkled on salads, oatmeal or added to smoothies. Chia seeds, since they make a jelly-like substance when added to liquid, are shown to pull toxins from the body.

Flax seeds

Flax seeds are high in protein and omega fatty acids. When these little seeds are consumed ground, they will digest better. Flax can be sprinkled on salads, oatmeal or added to smoothies.

Sunflower seeds

Sunflower seeds are a great snack on their own or added to a salad. These versatile seeds are tasty and full of vitamins and minerals to support healthy body function.

Pumpkin seeds

Pumpkin seeds are known to be high in zinc and other vitamins and minerals. These seeds are delicious raw and roasted and are the perfect addition to salads or as a simple grab-and-go snack.

Almonds

Almonds are known to be high in calcium, other minerals, vitamins, healthy fat and protein. Use these nuts as an addition to salads, to make raw desserts or plant-based milk.

Walnuts

Walnuts not only taste great but also rich in essential vitamins and minerals and heart-healthy unsaturated fats.

Cashews

Cashews are a high-fat, soft nut that make a perfect raw cheesecake, dairy-free cheese sauce, plant-based milk or healthy snack.

Coconut Flakes

Coconut is rich in healthy fat and the flakes make a great addition to oatmeal, cereal or smoothie.

Raw Cacao

Raw cacao is pure chocolate and very high in antioxidants, vitamins and minerals. This ingredient is perfect to have on hand for raw chocolates, desserts and warm beverages.

Nut butters

Nut butters can be used in a variety of recipes, spread on toast or used as a dip for fruit. My favourite nut butters to have on hand are peanut butter and almond butter.

Whole Grains & Flour

Whole grains are an important food for a well-balanced diet. Therefore, stocking your kitchen with a variety of whole-grains is essential for making a variety of healthy meals. Having a selection of flours available will allow you to make muffins or cookies when the mood strikes.

Some of the best whole grains and flour to have in your pantry include:

Brown, Black or Wild Rice

Rice is a gluten-free whole grain that can be used in a variety of ways. Eat alone, serve in a nori roll or with a vegetable stir-fry.

Quinoa

Quinoa is a gluten-free whole grain that is also very high in protein. It cooks faster than rice, can be used in sweet or savoury dishes and cold in salads.

Buckwheat

Buckwheat is a gluten-free grain that is a complete plant-based protein. It can be enjoyed as a breakfast cereal or addition to sweet or savoury dishes.

Whole-wheat flour

Organic whole-wheat flour can be used in baking and cooking a variety of dishes.

Almond meal

Almond meal is gluten-free flour that can be used in baking and cooking a variety of dishes.

Gluten-free flour

Many varieties of gluten-free flours are available and are perfect for people with gluten-intolerances or Celiac disease.

Teff

Teff is an ancient grain from Ethiopia and Eritrea. This whole grain is often ground into flour and used to make the traditional bread, which is a flat, pancake-like, fermented bread.

Plant-Based High-Protein Options

Tofu

Tofu is a food made from condensed soy milk that is pressed into solid white blocks. It originated in China, and the process is quite similar to how cheese is made. It is a good source of complete protein.

Tempeh

Tempeh is a fermented soy product high in protein, probiotics and a wide array of vitamins and minerals.

Lentils

Lentils are available in a variety of shapes and colours and are a versatile food. They are high in protein, fibre, vitamins and minerals.

Beans

Beans are high in protein and fibre. There are many different varieties of beans including: lima, black, black-eyed peas, kidney, garbanzo, kidney, navy and pinto.

Veggie burgers

Veggie burgers are one of my favourite dishes. You can make your own or buy delicious varieties to store in the freezer.

Vegan meat substitutes

Many delicious vegan meat substitutes are available. These meats include sausages, meatballs, burgers and more. Although, these meat substitutes are a processed food and for best health should only be eaten on occasion, they are nice to have on hand.

Oils

Having a variety of high-quality oils on-hand will allow you to cook with ease and make any homemade dressing in a flash. Although, it is nice to use oil in cooking and baking, you want to use them sparingly for best health.

Some of my favourite oils to keep in my pantry include:

Coconut oil

Coconut oil is very versatile and is considered a healthier source of plant-based saturated fat than animal saturated fat. It can be used to cook with, since it has a high tolerance to heat, and in raw dishes because it tastes great.

Olive oil

Olive oil is best used in raw dishes such as hummus or salad dressing. Be sure to purchase a high quality olive oil as some low-quality olive oils have been cut with other oils making it less heart-healthy.

Avocado oil

Avocado oil is a healthy source of unsaturated fat. This oil is a great replacement for olive oil in many salad dressings.

Peanut oil

Peanut oil can be used for frying as it can tolerate the heat. It is also a great addition to Asian-style cuisine.

Sunflower oil

Although this oil is not a necessity it works well in baking.

Spices

High-quality spices will either make or break a dish. Having a variety of spices in your pantry will give you the opportunity to change the flavour of any basic recipe.

Here are a few staple spices to have on-hand at all times:

Ground black pepper

Black pepper is one of the most common ingredients in cooking. You can choose a fine or course fresh ground.

147

Sea or Himalayan salt

Sea and Himalayan salts are the healthiest salts to consume. These salts are rich in essential minerals your body needs for optimal health.

Garlic powder

Garlic powder is made from dehydrating and grinding fresh garlic. It can be used a substitute for fresh garlic in any recipe and has a long shelf life.

Cumin

Cumin has a slightly nutty flavour and is a popular spice in dishes around the world including Mexican cuisine.

Coriander

Coriander is a nice spice to have on hand as international cuisine, such as Indian recipes, often call for its use.

Cardamom

Although this spice isn't as popular as some of the others I absolutely love its spicy, herbal and citrusy character. It goes well with cinnamon, nutmeg, clove, allspice and other aromatic spices.

Chili power

Chili powder is a spice blend that can be added to any chilli, taco or other dish you desire to have a little heat to it.

Cayenne pepper

Cayenne pepper is a very hot pepper used to flavour dishes of International cuisine. Keep cayenne in a shaker to add heat to any dish. This spice has also been shown to boost metabolism and have other health benefits.

Curry powder

Curry power is a blend of spices and often used in traditional Indian dishes.

Dried thyme

Thyme is a spice often popular in holiday-theme dishes. It is an intensely aromatic herb that goes well with any vegetable dish such as baked cauliflower or mushroom gravy. I will often substitute dried thyme with thyme essential oil.

Dried oregano

Oregano adds a subtle flavour to a dish and is typically used in Mexican and Italian cuisine. Like thyme, basil and cilantro having this spice in an essential oil form is a nice option to dried or fresh.

Dried basil

There are many varieties of fresh basil that make delicious additions to many dishes. However, having simple dried basil in your spice rack is an excellent replacement for fresh basil.

Dried rosemary

Rosemary is very aromatic and is a staple in a lot of Mediterranean and French cuisine. It has a woody and peppery quality that is very unique. Rosemary essential oil is a nice option as well.

Smoked (or regular) paprika

Paprika, especially the smoked version, adds a nice complexity to any dish. One of my favourite ways to use it is in dips or veggie pâté.

Cinnamon

Cinnamon can be used in both sweet and savoury dishes. This popular spice has been shown to help stabilize blood sugar and reduce blood cholesterol.

Ground ginger

Ground ginger has a warm spicy flavour and is most often used in baking but is also an important savoury ingredient used in International cuisine.

Cloves

This spice is often used in holiday baking, chai and barbecue rubs. Cloves are very strong and only need to be used in small quantities.

Turmeric

Turmeric is a spice that helps reduce inflammation and a delicious addition to savoury dishes and hot beverages. I like to add a teaspoon of turmeric powder or one drop of the essential oil to smoothies and savoury dishes.

Vanilla

Vanilla is a nice addition to all baking such as cookies and ice creams.

Condiments

Whether you have a plant-based kitchen or not, condiments are a staple. Although you may choose not to eat one or more of these condiments, pick your favourites to add them to your favourite dishes or snacks.

Nutritional yeast

Nutritional yeast is rich in vitamin B12 and has a cheesy-like flavour. Sprinkle on any salad or use it to make vegan cheese.

Ketchup

Ketchup is one of my favourite condiments. I am sure I eat potatoes just to eat ketchup. You can make your own or purchase an organic brand.

Mustard

Mustard is low in calories. It adds a nice zip to a burger, sausage or dressing and comes in many varieties.

Plant-based mayonnaise.

Follow Your Heart™ vegenaise is a plant-based mayonnaise. However, other brands are also available. This mayo makes a nice dip, addition to a burger or potato salad.

Maple syrup

Maple syrup is a delicious sugar substitute. Drizzle over fresh fruit or use in baking and salad dressings.

Apple cider vinegar

Apple cider vinegar can be used in salad dressings and other main dishes. It is also shown to have a variety of health benefits.

Barbecue sauce

Barbecue sauce adds a smokey zip to veggie

152

burgers, veggie sausages and other dishes. Make your own or buy an organic brand.

Supplements

As I've already mentioned in previous chapters, it's not easy to eat healthy every single day. We are busy and sometimes there's just not enough time to plan, prepare and make the healthiest meals.

When switching to a plant-based diet it is beneficial to use supplements and superfoods. Superfoods are nutritionally dense foods that will take enhance your health. Supplements and superfoods are not necessary for daily consumption but will help support good health especially on the days when your diet may not provide you with the nutrition you need.

Some the supplements and superfoods I recommend include:

Whole food fruit and veggie supplement

The reason I mention this one first is because no one in this modern world seems to eat enough fresh, ripe produce. The Canada Food Guide (2019) now recommends that half of each meal be made up of fruits and vegetables. That's a lot of eating and is not possible for many people.

I have been taking a whole food fruit and veggie supplement that contains the nutrients of over 30 different fruits and vegetables for many years. I have

153

more energy, experience faster recovery after my workouts and my skin is clear. This, in my opinion, is a staple in every kitchen.

Spirulina

Spirulina is blue-green algae. It is rich in protein and other healing properties. Although, it's technically a food you can buy it in a powder or capsules to take daily with your other supplements.

Wheatgrass

Wheatgrass is rich in chlorophyll, which is used by plants to absorb light energy. It has been shown to be extremely beneficial and healing to the body (Clement, 1998). Wheatgrass can be grown and juiced fresh. However; I like to buy dried wheatgrass powder and add it to smoothies or coconut water and take it with my other supplements.

Omega fatty acid blend

Omega fatty acids, especially omega-3 are essential for everyone to take to support good health (Greger, 2015). You can get omegas from food such as algae, hemp seeds, chia seeds and flax seeds but it is often easier to take a high-quality plant-based omega blend to ensure you are getting enough.

Vitamin B12 or B Complex

Vitamin B12 performs several key functions in the

154

body such as red blood cell formation, DNA synthesis, and supports neurological function. This vitamin comes from bacteria, not meat as it is often believed. Everyone, regardless of the kind of diet they choose to eat, needs enough vitamin B12 (Greger, 2015). When eating a plant-based diet, it is especially important to take a supplement that contains vitamin B12.

In a plant-focused diet, vitamin B12 can be obtained from eating fermented foods such as sauerkraut, kimchi and kombucha, as well as nutritional yeast. However, because many people do not eat enough of these foods, vitamin B12 intake can be scarce.

A Vitamin B complex supplement will give you a well-rounded intake of the B vitamins that play a vital role in the metabolism of carbohydrates, protein and fat.

Vitamin D3

If you live in Canada, or other countries further from the sun, it is important to take a vitamin D supplement daily (Greger, 2015).

Protein powder

One of the easiest ways to boost protein intake is to have a high-quality protein, or meal replacement, powder on hand. This can be simply added to any smoothie or blended with water to give a quick boost of protein throughout the day.

Superfoods

There are many superfoods and super herbs that can support and enhance your health that can be a great addition to your diet. For best results, please consult with a certified professional to learn about the best ones for your nutritional and health needs.

NOTE: Before taking any vitamin, mineral or other supplement(s) it is recommended that you check with your doctor and get blood tests first to be sure you are not taking something you don't need and you won't experience any negative side effects.

Chapter 9:
Meal Planning

Regardless of the type of diet you choose, it is important that you eat enough of the right nutrients. Earlier we discussed the serving size recommendations for macronutrients and the importance of eating a well-balanced diet.

Therefore, you will want to choose a variety of carbohydrates, fat and protein with each meal and take the recommended supplements to ensure you get all the nutrients you need for best health.

Why Meal Plan

Meal planning is important for a variety of reasons.

If you want to lose weight, meal planning will ensure you are getting the proper nutrients you need to fuel your body, rev up the metabolism to support weight loss without eating too little or too much.

If you want to have better fitness, performance and would like to be stronger and fitter, developing a meal plan will ensure you get the right amount of

157

proteins, carbs and fats in your diet as well as adequate pre and post workout nutrition.

If you are looking to simply gain better health, a meal plan will ensure you get a variety of whole food nutrition rich in the vitamins and minerals you need to support optimal health. Having a meal plan set out will also reduce the risk of eating too much junk or processed food.

Taking time to plan your meals is also a great way to practice mindful eating. When you take the time to determine the foods you will eat each week, pick up the items from the grocery store and prep the meals, you are developing a healthy relationship with food and you are actively involved in taking care of yourself and showing yourself self-love, which is key to better health and weight loss.

How To Plan Your Meals

Before you even get started with your specific meal plans for the week you will want to do these few things first:

1) Choose a day you will sit down and plan your meals for the week.

If you can get in the habit of choosing one day to do all of your planning it will be easier to get and stay in the habit.

2) Decide what and how much you are going to eat.

All you do in this step is simply take a moment to decide what you will eat though the week. You will want to make sure you are choosing a variety of foods and ones that support your goals. Figure out how much of each food you will eat each day that will support your personal goals and total it up for the week.

3) Go grocery shopping.

Now you get to go shopping. Some people love this part and others hate it. If you're someone who dislikes shopping for groceries, then I would suggest using a food delivery service. Many grocery stores have an online shopping system where you choose your items and the store personnel will gather the ingredients and deliver them to your home. It doesn't get much easier than that.

4) Make as many meals as you can.

Once you have your groceries organize them in a way that makes it easy for you to see what you have. Then, determine which items are for simple grab-and- go snacks and which ones will be for prepping meals. Prepare the quick snack items and store them in small bags or containers first. Next, prepare as many of the meals as you can and store in containers in the fridge or freezer until you're ready to eat them. Fresh, raw items such as salads may only

159

last two or three days before you have to make more. The more food you prepare ahead the more time you save each day, increasing your chances of staying on track with your goals.

5) Ensure you have the essential kitchen tools so you have what you need to make your meals.

Some of the essentials include, good set of knives, cutting board, food processor, blender, pots and pans and mixing bowls. Refer to chapter seven for more information on essential kitchen tools.

The Meal Planning Process

The first thing you will want to do when getting ready to plan your meals is to figure out your goals. Do you want to lose weight, gain weight, have more energy, gain strength, enhance endurance and athletic performance? It is essential to know your goals so you can develop the meal plan that suits your needs best.

If your desire is to lose weight, you will want to get an idea of how much and what kinds of foods you are eating now so you can change it to get the best results. The best way to do this is to write down everything you eat for two to three days during the week and one day on the weekend. Then, circle all the foods you think may not have been the healthiest choices, such as any processed or packaged foods, food high in saturated fat, fried foods, fast food and junk food.

160

Then, think about healthier options to replace these items with such as more fruits, veggies, legumes, whole grains, nuts and seeds, and the excess snacking, or meals, that can be cut out to reduce overall intake.

If you want to gain weight you can go through the same process but think about where you can add more healthy snacks or extra whole-food meals to add more calories to your diet.

If your goal is to increase performance, gain endurance and strength, support and speed up recovery after workouts you can go through a similar process but now focus on the timing of your meals. You want to be sure you're getting adequate nutrition before and after your workouts to support your performance.

In this meal planning process, you will learn how to develop a meal plan rich in whole-food plant-based nutrition, which will give you the results you're looking for regardless of your goals.

Components of a Healthy Diet

Before we get into meal planning we must first understand what makes up a healthy, plant-based diet. The updated Canada Food Guide (2019) suggests that:

- Half of the diet must consist of fresh fruits and veggies. There is ample evidence to show that a diet rich in fruits and veggies is the best way to support good health, reduce inflammation and as a result lose weight.

- A quarter of the diet should consist of whole grains. Whole grains have three parts, the endosperm, germ and bran. Whole grains provide the body with an abundance of fibre, vitamins such as the B vitamins and minerals such as iron and magnesium. It's best to stay away from all refined and process grains and carbohydrates as they contain little to no nutritional value and usually cause more harm than good.

- A quarter of the diet should consist of mostly plant proteins such as beans, lentils and peas. Of course these foods also contain healthy complex carbohydrates that provide fibre, vitamins and minerals.

You will also notice the glass in the Canada Food Guide is filled with water as water. It is essential to drink enough water to prevent dehydration and allow healthy body function to occur.

Use this equation to determine how much water you should drink for your body:

Body weight in pounds/2 = water in ounces
Water in ounces/8 = water in cups
Water in cups/4 = water in litres

You can also look at diet another way and that is by looking at your macronutrients, which are the bulk food that gives the body energy or helps it recover and repair. These are proteins, carbs and fats. I prefer to meal plan by using the plate theory such as the Canada Food Guide as it's an easier way to learn to eat intuitively. However, refer back to chapter six for the recommended macronutrient breakdown for best health.

Types Of Food To Include In Your Meal Plan

Is the previous section you learned about some basics of setting up your diet but here we will talk about some specific foods to include in your meal plan.

You already know that the bulk of your diet should come from fresh vegetables and fruit as well as whole grains, legumes, nuts and seeds.

You can choose from vegetables such as:

Fibrous vegetables:
- Asparagus
- Beets
- Bok choy
- Brussels sprouts
- Carrots
- Cucumbers
- Daikon radish
- Green beans
- Green peas

- Onions
- Sugar snap peas
- Squash, all varieties
- Tomatoes
- Watercress

Starchy vegetables:
- Parsnips
- Potatoes, white and sweet
- Pumpkin
- Squash
- Turnips
- Yams

Leafy greens:
- Beet greens
- Butter lettuce
- Collards
- Dandelion greens
- Kale, all varieties
- Lettuce, all varieties
- Spinach
- Swiss chard, all varieties

Sea vegetables:
- Agar
- Arame
- Dulse
- Kelp
- Kombu
- Nori
- Wake

As for fruit, you can pretty much choose any fruit but be aware some fruit will be higher in sugar than others. For example, berries, apples and pears are lower in sugar and your tropical fruits like mangoes, bananas and pineapple will be higher in sugar. Although all fruit contains natural sugars the body can use and fibre that helps keep to the blood sugar response low. It's best to consume fruits in their whole, raw form rather than as juice.

Fruit to choose from include:
- Apples
- Apricots
- Bananas
- Berries, all varieties
- Cherries
- Dates
- Dragon fruit
- Figs
- Grapefruit
- Grapes
- Kiwi
- Mangoes
- Melons
- Nectarines
- Oranges
- Papayas
- Peaches
- Pears
- Pineapple
- Plums
- Pomegranate

165

Legumes are your best source of plant-based protein as they also contain fibre and are low fat.

Legumes to choose include:
- Beans such as:
    - Adsuki
    - Black
    - Garbanzo (chickpeas)
    - Edamame
    - Fava
    - Kidney
    - Navy
    - Pinto
- Lentils such as:
    - Brown
    - Green
    - Red
- Peas such as:
    - Black-eyed
    - Green
    - Yellow
- Seitan
- Tempeh
- Tofu
- Veggie Burger

Another great source of protein in nutritional yeast. This is an inactive yeast that provides a flavour much like cheese to any dish.

Nuts and seeds are rich in protein as well as fat.

Nuts and seeds to choose include:
- Seeds such as:
    - Chia
    - Flax
    - Hemp
    - Pumpkin
    - Sesame
    - Sunflower
- Nuts such as:
    - Almonds
    - Brazil
    - Cashew
    - Hazelnuts
    - Macadamia
    - Pecans
    - Pine
    - Pistachios
    - Walnuts

Your complex carbs will come from fruit, veggies and legumes but it's also important to eat whole grains as a good source of complex carbohydrates.

Whole grains to choose include:
- Amaranth
- Buckwheat
- Millet
- Quinoa
- Rice, wild and brown
- Spelt
- Teff

A little oil will be ok in your meal plan as long as it's kept to a minimum.

Some oils to choose include:
- Coconut
- Flaxseed
- Hemp
- Olive, extra virgin
- Pumpkin seed

You will want to add a variety of herbs and spices to bring out the flavour in the food.

Some herbs and spices to include:
- Herbs:
    - Basil
    - Chilies
    - Cilantro
    - Dill
    - Mint
    - Oregano
    - Parsley
    - Thyme
- Spices:
    - Black pepper
    - Cardamon
    - Cayenne
    - Cinnamon
    - Cloves
    - Coriander
    - Cumin
    - Curry powder
    - Nutmeg

168

- Paprika
- Sea salt
- Turmeric

When developing a healthy meal plan you will want to keep sweets to a minimum but there's nothing wrong with indulging once in awhile.

Some sweeteners to have on hand include:
- Agave nectar
- Coconut nectar
- Maple syrup
- Stevia

Please refer to chapter eight for more suggested ingredients.

Sample Meal Plan

Now it's time for you to write out your meal plan. Start by taking a blank piece of paper and a pen, or use a software program such as Microsoft Excel™, Microsoft Word™ or iWork Pages™ programs to develop your meal plan.

Now, draw three columns and two rows and add these headings:

Breakfast	Mid Morning Snack	Lunch
Afternoon Snack	Dinner	Evening Snack

169

Next, fill out what you will have for each meal on a very basic level. Let's start with the macronutrients in order of importance for each meal.

Please remember this is only a sample. You will want to adjust to suit your own personal needs.

- Breakfast: complex carbohydrate, protein, fat.
- Mid-morning snack: carb, fat, protein,
- Lunch: protein, carb
- Afternoon snack: Protein/carb, or protein/ fat
- Dinner: Protein, carb, fat
- Evening snack: Carb, protein, fat

From here, add the carbohydrates, proteins and fats you want for your meals.

For example:
- Breakfast: oatmeal, 1/2 cup berries, 1 tsp hemp seeds, 1 tsp chia seeds, Mid-morning snack: low-fat coconut yogurt, 1/4 cup walnuts, 1/2 cup blueberries
- Lunch: 3 slices tempeh, 1/2 cup quinoa, tossed salad
- Afternoon snack: 1/2 cup roasted chickpeas, apple
- Dinner: tofu scramble with sweet potatoes and lots of veggies
- Evening snack: fruit, veggie smoothie with a scoop of protein powder

This is a simple example and one you can use to design your meal plan for each day of the week.

Below is another sample meal plan that includes a variety of recipes for you to try. Use this meal plan as a guide but feel free to adjust it to suit your taste and lifestyle. Be creative and have fun!

As you will notice, this plan includes a variety of mostly cooked meal options to help you adjust to this type of food. As you become more familiar with a plant-based diet you may choose to embrace a more raw, and super food rich diet to take your health to the next level.

Sample Meal Plan				
Day	**Breakfast**	**Lunch**	**Snack**	**Dinner**
Sunday	Mediterranean tofu scramble	TLT sandwich	Spicy hummus & veggies	Coconut Thai vegetable soup
Monday	Banana split smoothie	Sweet & spicy roasted vegetables	Oatmeal & raisin square	Veggie burger with tossed salad
Tuesday	Toast with organic peanut butter & jam	Leftover roasted vegetables	Tropical green smoothie	Chick'n kale caesar salad
Wednesday	Blueberry bliss smoothie	Quinoa salad	Handful of nuts and raw veggies	Veggie chili
Thursday	Granola with almond milk	Leftover quinoa salad	Guacamole with organic tortilla chips or veggies	Pad Thai
Friday	Very berry smoothie	Leftover veggie chili	Oatmeal & Raisin Square	Stuffed portobello mushroom & tossed salad
Saturday	Oatmeal & fruit	Sea & sun pâté with veggies & crackers	Chocolate pudding	Pasta with red pepper marinara & meatless meatballs

All these recipes, and more, are found in the next chapter.

Chapter 10:
Recipes

This chapter includes a collection of my own recipe creations. Use these recipes to create your own meal plan based on what you learned in the last chapter.

Recipes:

A BEGINNERS GUIDE TO GOING MEATLESS

Banana Split Smoothie

Ingredients:
- 1 banana
- 1 cup strawberries
- 1 cup coconut milk
- 2 tbsp. cacao powder
- 1 tbsp. chia seeds
- 1 tbsp. hemp seeds
- Optional: 1 scoop chocolate plant-based protein powder

Instructions:
- Place all ingredients in a high-speed blender.
- Blend until smooth.

Barbecue Jackfruit Hawaiian Pizza

Ingredients for crust:
- 2 heads cauliflower
- 1 garlic head
- 2 tbsp. coconut oil, melted
- 3 tbsp. ground flaxseed + 8 tbsp. water
- ½ tsp. sea salt
- 6 tbsp. nutritional yeast
- 2 tsp. dried oregano
- 2 tsp. dried basil
- 2 tbsp. arrowroot starch
- 2 ½ cups organic whole grain flour

Ingredients for pizza toppings:
- ½ small can of tomato sauce
- 1-2 tbsp. dried oregano
- 1 small onion, diced
- ½ red pepper, diced
- 1 package barbecue jackfruit
- ½ cup fresh pineapple, chopped
- 1 package Daiya™ cheese shreds

Instructions:
- Preheat oven to 375°F.
- Wash and roughly chop up cauliflower to bite size pieces. Peel the outside of the head of garlic.
- Place cauliflower and garlic on a greased baking pan. Drizzle with coconut oil.
- Bake for 30 minutes or until soft and allow to cool.

177

- Remove garlic cloves from skin and pull cauliflower apart and place both in a food processor. Process until smooth.
- Separately, place the flax and water mixture in a large bowl and allow to set.
- Add salt, oregano, basil and arrow root starch and stir until mixed.
- Add flour a little at a time until doughy consistency achieved.
- Place parchment paper on a pizza pan.
- Lightly dust the dough with flour and spread out with hands or a small rolling pin to the edges.
- Bake for 40 minutes.
- Flip and bake for 10 more minutes.
- Spread tomato sauce evenly on crust and sprinkle oregano on top.
- Add remaining toppings and bake for 10 minutes or until browned on top and sides.
- Optional: Broil for 2 minutes to crisp the cheese.

Blueberry Bliss Smoothie

Ingredients:
- 1 ½ cups fresh or frozen blueberries
- 1 banana
- 1 handful spinach
- 1 tbsp. hemp seed
- 1 cup coconut milk
- Optional: 1 scoop vanilla plant-based protein powder.

Instructions:
- Place all ingredients into a high-speed blender.
- Blend until smooth.

Chick'n Kale Caesar Salad

Dressing ingredients:
- ¼ cup cashews, soaked for at least 1 hour
- ¼ cup pine nuts, soaked for at least 1 hour
- 1 tbsp. miso paste (any kind will do)
- 2 tbsp. nutritional yeast
- 4 cloves garlic
- 2 tbsp. olive oil
- 1 lemon, juiced
- 1 tbsp. balsamic vinegar
- 1 date, pitted
- ½ tsp. ground cumin
- Pinch of sea salt
- ¼ cup water

Salad ingredients:
- 2 cups chopped romaine lettuce
- 2 cups kale, chopped
- 1 cucumber, chopped
- 1 red pepper, chopped
- 1 large carrot, grated
- ½ red onion, chopped
- 1 package Gardein™ meatless chick'n strips, cooked according to instructions

Instructions:
- Mix all dressing ingredients in a blender until smooth and set aside.
- While cooking the chick'n strips, prepare the salad.

- When the chick'n strips are cooked, pour the dressing over the salad and mix until everything is covered with dressing.
- To serve, place two cups of salad on a plate, place chick'n strips on top and serve with a toasted baguette.

Chickpea Salad Sandwich

Ingredients:
- 1 small can chickpeas, drained and rinsed
- 2-3 tbsp. red onion, finely diced
- 2-3 tbsp. Follow Your Heart™ original vegenaise
- 2-3 tbsp. dill pickle, diced into very small pieces
- 1 celery stalk, diced
- 1 tbsp. mustard
- 1 tsp. turmeric
- ½ tsp. sea salt
- 4 slices whole-grain or gluten-free bread
- 2 lettuce leaves
- 4 slices tomato
- Sea salt to taste
- Black pepper to taste
- Garlic powder to taste

Instructions:
- Place all ingredients, except bread, lettuce leaves and tomato, into a food processor and process until thoroughly mixed but still chunky.
- Set aside.
- Lightly toast bread and top with lettuce and tomato.
- Add chickpea salad mixture and serve as an open or closed-face sandwich.

Chocolate Macaroons

Ingredients:
- 3 cups dried, shredded organic coconut flakes
- ⅓ cup coconut oil, melted
- 1 cup raw cacao powder
- 1 tbsp. vanilla powder
- ½ tsp. sea salt
- 1 cup maple syrup

Instructions:
- In a large bowl, combine all the ingredients in the order listed and stir well to combine.
- Prepare a cookie sheet lined with parchment paper.
- Using a small melon baller, spoon rounds of the mixture onto a cookie sheet dehydrator sheet.
- Refrigerate until cookies are solid.

Chocolate Pudding

Ingredients:
- 1 avocado
- 1 banana
- ½ cup coconut water, at room temperature (or more if needed to thin)
- 4 tbsp. raw cacao powder
- 1 tbsp. vanilla powder
- 1 tbsp. chia seeds
- ¼ tsp. sea salt

Instructions:
- In a high-speed blender, puree all ingredients until completely smooth, stopping to scrape the sides as necessary.
- Transfer to bowls and chill for a firmer pudding, or consume immediately.
- Serve with raspberries and fresh mint or chopped nuts.

Coconut Thai Vegetable Soup

Ingredients:
- 1 small can (400 mL) coconut milk
- 3 cups vegetable broth
- 3 tbsp. green curry paste
- 2 tbsp. Bragg's™ liquid aminos
- 2 cups broccoli, chopped
- 2 cups zucchini, chopped
- 3 celery sticks, chopped
- 1 large yellow carrot, chopped
- 1 tbsp. maple syrup
- ¼ tsp. sea salt
- 1 tbsp. lime juice
- ¼ cup cilantro, chopped
- 1 tbsp. hemp seeds

Instructions:
- Add coconut milk, vegetable broth, green curry paste and Bragg's™ liquid aminos to a large pot and bring to a boil.
- Reduce heat and add broccoli, zucchini, carrot, celery, maple syrup, sea salt and lime juice.
- Simmer on low for about five minutes.
- Place in bowls; top with cilantro and hemp seeds and serve.

Cucumber Rolls

Ingredients for sauce:
- ½ cup almond butter
- ½ tbsp. fresh ginger, chopped
- 2 tbsp. lemon juice
- ½ tsp. sea salt

Ingredients for rolls:
- 1-2 cucumbers sliced lengthwise
- 1 carrot, cut in half and sliced julienne style
- handful broccoli sprouts
- 10 or more basil leaves
- 10 or more mint leaves

Instructions:
- Blend all ingredients for the sauce and set aside.
- Place cucumber strips on a cutting board or plate.
- Spread out almond sauce on each slice of cucumber.
- Top with one carrot stick placed across the cucumber, a small pinch of sprouts, one basil leaf and one mint leaf.
- Roll up the cucumber from one end to the other like a sushi roll.
- Place a toothpick in the centre to hold together.

Guacamole

Ingredients:
- 3 avocados, peeled and pitted
- 1 lime, or lemon, juiced
- 1 tsp. sea salt
- ½ cup onion, diced
- 1 clove garlic, minced
- 2 Roma tomatoes, diced
- 3 tbsp. fresh cilantro, chopped

Instructions:
- Place avocado in a mixing bowl with the lime or lemon juice and mash until desired consistency is reached.
- Add remaining ingredients and stir until fully mixed.
- Serve with raw veggies and crackers.

Kale Salad

Ingredients:
- 1 head curly green kale, washed, dried, stems removed, and chopped
- 1 avocado
- ½ lemon, juiced
- 1 tbsp. cold pressed olive oil
- 1 tomato
- 1 cucumber, peeled and chopped
- 1 date, chopped
- ½ cup cranberries
- 1 tbsp. hemp seeds
- pinch of sea salt

Instructions:
- Place kale, salt, lemon juice and olive oil in a bowl. Massage kale leaves until they become a little softer and are fully coated.
- Set aside.
- Add remaining ingredients to the bowl.
- Toss and serve.
- Store leftovers in a sealed glass container for two or three days.

Key Lime Mousse

Ingredients:
- ¾ cup avocado, mashed
- ¼ cup maple syrup
- 2 tbsp. lime juice

Instructions:
- Place all ingredients in a blender or food processor and mix until smooth.
- Scoop into martini glass and enjoy.

Lemon Lentil Power Bowl

Ingredients for bowl:
- 1 cup brown rice
- 1 cup black lentils
- 4 cups water (2 cups for rice & 2 cups for lentils)
- 1 tbsp. coconut oil
- ½ red onion
- 3 garlic cloves, crushed
- 8 sun dried tomatoes
- 1 red or yellow pepper
- ¼ tsp. salt
- ¼ tsp. black pepper
- 2 handfuls spinach
- 1 tomato, chopped
- ⅓ bunch parsley

Ingredients for lemon tahini dressing:
- ¼ cup tahini, raw
- ¾ cup lemon or lime juice, fresh
- ¼ cup nutritional yeast
- ½ cup raw cashews
- ⅔ cup water
- 1 tbsp. garlic, minced
- 1 tsp. sea salt
- 1 tsp. black pepper

Instructions:
- Place rice and two cups of water in a medium to large pot and cover with lid.
- Bring to a boil, reduce heat and simmer for 40 minutes until cooked.

- At the same time, place lentils and two cups of water in a medium to large pot and cover with lid.
- Bring to a boil, reduce heat and simmer for 40 minutes until cooked and all water is absorbed.
- Place all dressing ingredients into a high-speed blender, blend until thoroughly mixed and set aside.
- In a large pan, heat coconut oil over medium heat.
- Add onion, garlic, sun dried tomatoes, peppers, salt, and pepper, stir and cook until soft.
- Add rice and lentils. Stir until mixed.
- Add tahini dressing and stir.
- Allow to heat up for up to five minutes.
- Add spinach, tomatoes and parsley and stir until mixed.
- Once spinach has slightly wilted scoop into bowls and serve.
- Store this dish in a sealed glass container and refrigerate for up to five days.
- This dish is delicious served cold, or heated, on a bed of spinach or lettuce.

Lentil & Veggie Soup

Ingredients:
- 1 tbsp. coconut oil
- 2 large carrots, chopped
- 1 large onion, chopped
- 1 zucchini, chopped
- 4 cloves garlic, minced
- 6 cups water or vegetable broth
- 1 cup green lentils
- 1 celery stalk, chopped
- 5 fresh ripe tomatoes, chopped
- 1 tbsp. dried basil
- 1 ½ tsp. sea salt
- ½ tsp. fresh ground pepper
- ¼ cup Italian parsley, chopped

Instructions:
- Heat oil in a large soup pot.
- Add carrots, onion and zucchini and sauté on medium heat until soft (about 4 to 5 minutes).
- Add garlic and sauté two or three minutes longer.
- Add all remaining ingredients except parsley.
- Bring to a boil, reduce heat and simmer for 45 to 50 minutes, or until lentils are tender. Stir occasionally.
- When ready, serve in a nice bowl and garnish with parsley.
- Store in glass container for up to five days.

Lentil Dahl

Ingredients:
- 1 tsp. coconut oil
- 1 sweet onion, diced
- 3 garlic cloves, minced
- 1 tbsp. fresh ginger, finely minced
- ½ tsp. red chili flakes
- 2 tsp. ground turmeric
- 1 tsp. garam masala or other curry powder blend
- ½ tsp. ground cumin
- ½ tsp. ground coriander
- ½ tsp. ground mustard
- 1 cup dried red lentils, uncooked
- 1 can (400 ml) diced tomatoes
- 1 can (400 ml) coconut milk
- 2 cups vegetable broth
- ⅛ tsp. salt
- ⅛ tsp. pepper
- Juice of half a lemon
- 2 cups fresh spinach

Instructions:
- Heat oil in a large pot over medium heat.
- Add onion and cook for up to five minutes.
- Add garlic, ginger, red chili, turmeric, garam masala, cumin, coriander and mustard. Stir until mixed and cook for one minute.
- Add lentils, tomatoes, coconut milk and vegetable broth. Cover, bring to a boil and cook on medium to low heat for 15 to 20 minutes.
- Add lemon juice and spinach. Stir until spinach wilts then serve on a bed of rice.

Mango Coconut Chia Pudding

Ingredients:
- 1 cup coconut milk
- ¾ cup fresh or frozen mangoes, diced (if using frozen be sure to thaw first)
- 2 tbsp. chia seeds
- 1 tbsp. sweetened shredded coconut
- 1 tsp. maple syrup

Instructions:
- Combine all ingredients in a large glass jar.
- Mix well and seal.
- Refrigerate for at least five to six hours before serving.

Mediterranean Tofu Scramble

Ingredients:
- 1 tbsp. coconut oil
- ½ cup sweet onion, diced
- 1 garlic clove, minced
- ½ cup bell pepper, diced
- ½ cup zucchini, diced
- 3 crimini mushrooms, chopped
- ¼ cup sun dried tomatoes
- 1 large block organic extra firm tofu, crumbled
- 2 tbsp. fresh basil, chopped
- 1 tbsp. turmeric
- 1 tbsp. Bragg's™ Liquid Soy Seasoning
- 1 handful spinach

Instructions:
- Place coconut oil in a medium frying pan over medium heat.
- As you prepare the ingredients, in the order they are listed, add them to the pan, stirring occasionally.
- When warm remove from heat and enjoy!

Oatmeal Raisin Squares

Ingredients:
- 1 tbsp. coconut oil
- 5 medium sweet potatoes, washed, peeled and diced into cubes.
- 4 cups quick oats
- ¾ cup almond milk mixed with 1 tbsp. lemon juice
- ¼ cup ground flaxseed
- ½ cup maple syrup
- 1 tbsp. cinnamon
- 1 tbsp. nutmeg
- ½ cup raisins
- ½ cup raw, unsalted almonds, chopped
- pinch sea salt

Instructions:
- Preheat oven to 400°F.
- Lightly coat a baking pan with coconut oil.
- Place potatoes in baking pan and place in the oven for 20 minutes, stir and cook for another 20 minutes until tender.
- Remove from the oven and cool.
- When cool, place in a mixing bowl. Add remaining ingredients and mix well.
- Press into a lightly greased baking pan and bake for 30 to 35 minutes or until lightly golden on top.
- Remove from heat, cool, cut into squares and serve.

Pasta with Red Pepper Marinara & Meatless Meatballs

Ingredients for pasta:
- ½ to 1 package of whole grain, non-GMO pasta, cooked according to instructions
- One package of Gardein™ meatless meatballs

Ingredients for sauce:
- 1 red bell pepper, chopped
- ½ red onion, chopped
- 1 bunch fresh basil, chopped
- 1 clove garlic
- 1 tbsp. Bragg's™ liquid aminos
- 1 tbsp. oregano
- ½ tbsp. rosemary
- ½ cup extra virgin olive oil
- 1 tsp. fresh lemon juice
- fresh thyme to taste
- 1 tbsp. maple syrup
- 1 tbsp. nutritional yeast

Instructions:
- In a food processor, combine all sauce ingredients and process to a fine texture.
- Pour into a small saucepan and heat on low to medium heat.
- Cook meatless meatballs according to instructions and add to sauce to simmer.
- Top pasta with sauce and meatless meatballs.
- Serve with a fresh baguette topped with coconut oil, a sprinkle of nutritional yeast and fresh garlic or a sprinkle of garlic powder.

197

Pad Thai

Ingredients for sauce:
* ½ cup almond butter
* ½ cup sun dried tomatoes, soaked for 2 hours
* 1 lime, chopped
* 4 cloves garlic, peeled
* 7 dates, pitted
* ¼ cup olive oil
* 1 jalapeño, chopped
* 1 ½ tbsp. ginger, shredded
* 1 tbsp. Bragg's™ liquid aminos or tamari sauce
* 1 tsp. sea salt

Ingredients for pad Thai:
* 1-package rice pad Thai noodles or zucchini for raw version
* 1 tbsp. coconut oil
* ½ sweet onion, diced
* 2 garlic cloves
* 1 red bell pepper, diced
* 10 sugar snap peas, chopped
* 1 cup almonds, chopped
* ¼ cup cilantro
* 2 large handfuls bean sprouts

Instructions:
* Place all sauce ingredients in blender and mix until smooth.
* Place in a saucepan and heat on low to medium heat until warm, set aside.
* Cook rice noodles according to instructions.

198

- Place onion and garlic in skillet with coconut oil and sauté for two to three minutes.
- Add pepper and sugar snap peas and sauté for another two to three minutes.
- Place rice noodles and bean sprouts in a large bowl.
- Pour sauce over noodles and toss until all noodles are covered.
- Top with almonds and cilantro and serve.

199

Parsnip Fries

Ingredients:
- 4 large parsnips
- 2 tbsp. coconut oil
- 1 tsp. sea salt or truffle sea salt
- 1 tsp. oregano
- 1 tsp. rosemary

Instructions:
- Preheat oven to 400°F.
- Peel the parsnips and cut them julienne (french fry) style.
- Mix parsnips with the remaining ingredients in a bowl and spread out onto cookie sheet.
- Bake for 10 to 15 minutes until golden.

Peanut Butter Chocolate Chip Cookies

Ingredients:
- ½ cup Earth's Balance Vegan Butter
- 1 cup sugar
- 1 tbsp. vanilla extract
- 3 tbsp. coconut milk
- 1 cup peanut butter
- 1 & ½ cups organic, unbleached all purpose flour
- 1 tsp. baking soda
- ½ tsp. sea salt
- ¾ cup small dairy-free chocolate chips

Instructions:
- Preheat oven to 375°F.
- Place coconut oil, sugar, vanilla and coconut milk in a large bowl. Use a hand mixer to mix until creamy.
- Add peanut butter and mix until well combined.
- In a separate bowl mix flour, baking soda and salt.
- Add dry ingredients to wet ingredients and used your hands, or spatula, until you get a thick, crumbly dough. If dough is too dry add a touch of coconut milk.
- Add chocolate chips and mix thoroughly.
- Roll into balls, about 1 tbsp. per ball, and place on a parchment lined baking sheet.
- Bake for 15 minutes until tops are golden brown. Remove from heat and allow cookies to cool and firm up on the baking sheet before moving them to a cool surface.

Peanut Tofu Bowl

Ingredients:
- 1 tsp. coconut oil
- ½ sweet onion, diced
- 1 cup frozen mixed vegetables
- 2, 350 gram blocks of tofu, drained and cut into 1-inch pieces
- 1 cup broccoli, cut into bite sized pieces
- ½ cup creamy organic peanut butter
- 1 cup full fat coconut milk
- 2 tbsp. Bragg's™ soy sauce
- 2 tbsp. maple syrup
- 1 tbsp. sriracha
- 2 tsp. fresh ginger, finely minced
- 2 cloves garlic, minced
- Juice of 1 lime

Instructions:
- Heat oil in large pan on medium heat. Add onion and frozen mixed vegetables and sauté until soft; about five minutes.
- Add tofu and sauté until browned.
- Add broccoli. Reduce to low until peanut sauce is ready.
- For sauce: add peanut butter, coconut milk, Bragg's™, maple syrup, sriracha, ginger, garlic and lime to a small pot on medium to low heat.
- Whisk often until smooth and creamy, about five to 10 minutes.
- Add sauce to tofu and vegetables and stir to coat each piece.
- Serve over a bed of rice.

Pineapple Curry Stir-Fry

Ingredients for stir-fry:
- 1 cup brown rice
- 2 cups vegetable broth
- 3 tbsp. organic coconut oil
- 1 medium sweet onion, diced
- 2 large celery stalks, chopped
- 2 large carrots, diced
- 1 head of broccoli, chopped
- ½ head green cabbage, chopped
- ½ head cauliflower, chopped
- 2 inch pieces of fresh ginger (or 1 tsp. ground ginger)
- 6 cloves of fresh garlic, minced
- 2 cups chickpeas (soaked and cooked from dry, otherwise use one 450 mL can)
- 1 cup fresh or frozen pineapple, diced

Ingredients for coconut curry dressing:
- 1 cup organic coconut milk, canned
- 1 cup organic vegetable stock (or more if desired)
- 4 tbsp. mild curry powder
- sea salt and fresh ground pepper to taste.

Instructions for veggies:
- Place one cup brown rice and two cups vegetable broth in a large covered pot bring to a boil over high heat.
- Reduce heat to low. Simmer until lentils are soft and all liquid is absorbed.

- In a large skillet heat coconut oil over medium-high heat.
- Add onion and celery and allow to cook, stirring occasionally for about five minutes.
- Add all remaining ingredients except pineapple.
- Stir until thoroughly heated.
- Add pineapple and stir occasionally until warm.

Instructions for sauce:
- Place all ingredients in a high-speed blender until thoroughly mixed.
- Adjust salt, pepper and curry powder until desired taste achieved.
- Pour sauce over veggies and simmer until warm.

Instructions for stir-fry:
- Place one to two cups of brown rice in a bowl.
- Top with one to two cups of veggies in sauce.

Pumpkin Spice Tart

Ingredients for crust:
- 2 cups unsweetened flaked coconut
- 2 ½ cups raw walnuts
- ¾ tsp. salt
- 1 ¼ cup dates, pitted
- 1 tsp. cinnamon
- 1 tbsp. filtered water, added as needed

Ingredients for filling:
- 2 cups raw cashews, soaked 2 hours or more
- 2 cups carrot juice, freshly juiced
- ¼ cup agave nectar
- ¾ cup coconut oil
- ½ cup fresh dates, pitted
- 1 tbsp. cinnamon
- 1 tsp. vanilla extract
- 2 tsp. ground ginger
- ½ tsp. ground nutmeg
- ¼ tsp. ground cloves
- ¾ tsp. sea salt

Instructions:
- Place all crust ingredients, except water, in food processor until moist and sticky.
- Add water if necessary to bind the mixture.
- Spoon one tablespoon of mixture into each space of a mini muffin tin.
- Press firmly, coating the bottom and sides of the cups.
- Place in the freezer until you make the filling.

- Place all filling ingredients in a high-speed blender and blend until smooth.
- Pour into muffin tin cups.
- Chill for two hours or more until set before serving.

Quinoa Salad

Ingredients:
- 4 cups quinoa, cooked
- 4 green onions, thinly chopped
- 1 large tomato, seeded and finely diced
- ¾ English cucumber, peeled and chopped
- ¼ cup parsley, minced
- 4 tbsp. extra virgin olive oil
- 5 tbsp. lemon juice
- 2 tbsp. Bragg's™ liquid aminos
- ½ tsp. fennel seed

Instructions:
- Mix everything in a large bowl.
- Serve immediately or let sit for one hour to allow the flavours to meld together.

Rainbow Slaw Salad

Ingredients for salad:
- 1 bell pepper, sliced julienne
- 1 large carrot, sliced julienne
- 1 zucchini, sliced julienne
- 1 beet, sliced julienne
- 1 apple, sliced julienne
- 2 cloves garlic, minced
- 2 tbsp. fresh ginger, minced
- ½ cup chopped walnuts
- ½ cup raisins
- ¼ cup fresh mint, chopped
- ½ cup fresh basil, chopped
- ½ bunch fresh cilantro, chopped

Ingredients for dressing:
- ½ cup lemon juice, freshly squeezed
- ½ cup olive oil
- 1 clove garlic, minced
- 1 tbsp. fresh ginger, minced
- 1 tbsp. tamari, or soy sauce
- 1 tbsp. maple syrup

Instructions:
- Place all salad ingredients in a large bowl.
- Place all dressing ingredients into a high-speed blender and blend until smooth.
- Pour desired amount of dressing over salad and serve.

Sea & Sun Pâté

Ingredients:
- 2 sheets nori
- 1 large garlic clove
- ¾ cup sunflower seeds
- 1 ½ inch green onion, cut from bottom
- 1 celery stalk, chopped
- 1 large carrot, grated
- ½ cup parsley,
- 3 tbsp. olive oil
- 2 tbsp. Bragg's™ liquid aminos
- 1 ½ tbsp. nutritional yeast
- 1 tsp. cumin
- 1 tsp. paprika
- 4 tbsp. black sesame seeds (optional)
- 4 tbsp. white sesame seeds (optional)

Instructions:
- Mix nori, garlic, sunflower seeds, onion, and celery in a food processor and blend until roughly mixed.
- Add remaining ingredients, except sesame seeds, and process until thoroughly mixed but still slightly chunky.
- Top with sesame seeds and serve with sliced cucumbers or crackers.

Shepherd's Pie

Ingredients for mashed potatoes:
- 6-8 large potatoes, wash, peeled and diced
- 3-4 tbsp. coconut oil
- ¼ - ½ cup coconut milk, add more if needed
- pinch of salt and pepper, to taste

Ingredients for filling:
- 1 ½ cups uncooked brown or green lentils
- 3 cups vegetable broth
- 1 tbsp. coconut oil
- 1 medium onion, diced
- 2 cloves garlic, minced
- 1 celery stalk, chopped
- 2 cups frozen peas and carrots
- 1 bag gluten-free Gardein™ beefless ground
- 1 ½ tsp. dried thyme
- ¼ tsp. sea salt
- ¼ tsp. black pepper
- ½ tsp. garlic powder
- 1-2 tbsp. nutritional yeast

Instructions:
- Place potatoes in a large pot and fill with water until covered.
- Bring to a boil on high heat, reduce to medium-high heat, cover and cook for 20 to 30 minutes or until soft.
- While the potatoes are cooking place lentils and vegetable stock in a medium pot.
- Cover and bring to a boil.
- Reduce heat and simmer until all vegetable

broth has been absorbed and lentils are soft.

- While potatoes and lentils are cooking, preheat oven to 425°F and lightly grease a 9x13 pan.
- In a large saucepan over medium heat, sauté onions, garlic and celery in coconut oil until lightly browned and caramelized (about five minutes).
- Add frozen vegetables and Gardein™ beefless ground.
- Cook, stirring occasionally until veggies are soft.
- Add thyme, salt, pepper and garlic powder adjusting to taste.
- Add cooked lentils and thoroughly mix with the beefless ground and veggies.
- Place filling in a prepared oven-safe baking dish and flatten into the pan with a spatula.
- Once potatoes are cooked, drain and place back in the pot.
- Add coconut oil and coconut milk.
- Using a masher, or hand mixer mash until smooth. Add more coconut milk as needed until desired consistency is achieved (add slowly to prevent using too much).
- Season with salt and pepper to taste and set aside.
- Carefully top with mashed potatoes and smooth with a spatula.
- Top with a sprinkle of nutritional yeast.
- Place in the oven and bake for 20 to 30 minutes or until the mashed potatoes are lightly browned on top.

- Let cool briefly before serving. The longer it sits, the more it will thicken.
- Before covering and storing in the fridge, allow it to completely cool.
- Keeps up to five days and reheats well in the oven or pan.

Spicy Hummus

Ingredients:
- 1, 540 ml can chickpeas
- ¼ cup olive oil
- Juice of 1 lime
- 1 clove garlic, minced
- 1 tsp. salt
- 1 tsp. ground cumin
- 1 tsp. ground coriander
- ½ tsp. cracked pepper
- ¼ tsp. cayenne
- pinch turmeric

Instructions:
- Mix all ingredients in a food processor or blender until smooth.
- Serve with raw veggies or crackers.

Stuffed Portobello Mushrooms

Ingredients:
- 1 tbsp. coconut oil
- 4 medium Portobello mushrooms
- 2 cloves garlic, minced
- ½ small sweet onion, chopped
- 2 cups spinach leaves
- 1 ½ cups cooked chickpeas
- 1 tbsp. almond flour
- 1 tbsp. water
- ½ tsp. ground coriander
- ½ tsp. cumin
- ¼ tsp. sea salt
- ¼ tsp. ground black pepper

Instructions:
- Preheat oven to 425°F.
- Grease a baking sheet with coconut oil.
- Scrape out the inside gills of the mushrooms and place on the cookie sheet.
- Place remaining ingredients in a food processor and process until mixed but not too smooth.
- Place one quarter of the mixture in each mushroom cap and bake for 20 minutes or until filling is golden brown on the top.

Sweet and Spicy Roasted Veggies

Ingredients:
- 1 large sweet potato, diced
- 1 red bell pepper, diced
- 2 cups mushrooms, diced
- 1 sweet onion, chopped
- 2 tomatoes, chopped
- 1 cup Brussels sprouts
- 2 large carrots, chopped
- 2 large parsnips, chopped
- 1, 400 mL can pineapple chunks
- 3 tbsp. coconut oil
- 2 garlic cloves, pressed
- 1 tsp. dill weed
- 1 tsp. sea salt
- 1 ½ tsp. cayenne pepper
- 1 ½ tsp. garlic powder
- 1 tsp. fresh ground pepper

Instructions:
- Preheat oven to 350°F.
- Place all ingredients in a large roaster.
- Mix well.
- Cover and place in oven.
- Stir veggies every ten minutes until soft.

TLT Sandwich

Ingredients:
- 2 slices of vegan bread
- 1 tbsp. coconut oil
- 2-4 tempeh strips
- ½ avocado
- ½ tomato, sliced
- 1-2 leaves of lettuce
- ¼ cup sprouts
- 1 tbsp. Follow Your Heart™ original vegenaise
- 1 tbsp. Dijon mustard
- Sea salt, to taste
- Black pepper, to taste
- Garlic powder, to taste

Instructions:
- Place tempeh strips in a frying pan on medium to low heat with coconut oil and cook each side until golden brown.
- Toast the bread.
- Spread mayo on one side of the toast and mustard on the other.
- Place avocado, tomatoes, lettuce, sprouts and tempeh on the toast.
- Serve with soup or salad.

Tropical Green Smoothie

Ingredients:
- 1 banana, frozen
- 1 orange, peeled
- ½ cup mangoes, frozen
- ½ cup pineapple, frozen
- 1 handful spinach
- 2 cup almond milk
- ¼ tsp. vanilla bean powder or extract
- Optional: 1 scoop vanilla plant-based protein powder

Instructions:
- Place all ingredients into a high-speed blender.
- Blend until smooth.

Veggie Burger

Ingredients:
- 1 cup crimini mushrooms
- 1 cup wheat-free instant oats
- 1 small can organic black beans, drained
- ½ large sweet onion, chopped
- ¼ cup nutritional yeast
- 3 cloves garlic
- 2 tbsp. Bragg's™ Liquid Aminos
- 1 tbsp. ground chia seeds
- 1 tsp. ground black pepper
- ¼ tsp. sea salt
- 1 carrot, peeled and grated
- ½ zucchini, grated,
- ½ beet, peeled and grated

Instructions:
- Preheat oven to 375°F.
- Place parchment paper on a cookie sheet and grease with coconut oil.
- Place all ingredients, except carrot, zucchini and beet, in food processor and blend until thoroughly mixed. Set aside.
- Place mixture in a bowl and add the carrot, zucchini and beet.
- Thoroughly mix ingredients by hand.
- Form mixture into patties, place on the cookie sheet and bake for 12 minutes.
- Flip and bake another 10 minutes.
- Serve on a fresh whole grain or gluten-free bun with a tossed salad.

Veggie Chili

Ingredients:
- 3 tbsp. coconut oil
- 1 sweet onion, chopped
- ½ yellow pepper
- ½ red pepper
- ½ - 1 zucchini, chopped
- 5 cloves of garlic, pressed
- 4 fresh tomatoes, diced, or one large can of diced tomatoes
- ½ cup water
- 1 can sweet corn kernels
- 1 cup fresh mushrooms chopped
- 1 tbsp. maple syrup
- 1 tbsp. coriander
- 2 tsp. sea salt
- 2 ½ tsp. ground cumin
- 1 tsp. chili powder
- 1 small can organic chickpeas (garbanzo beans)
- 1 small can organic baked beans in tomato sauce
- 3 tbsp. nutritional yeast

Instructions:
- In a large pot heat coconut oil on medium-high heat.
- Add onion, peppers, Brussels sprouts, and garlic.
- Cook three to five minutes stirring as needed.

219

- Add tomatoes, water, corn, mushrooms, maple syrup, coriander, sea salt, cumin, and chili powder.
- Reduce heat to medium-low.
- Add beans and nutritional yeast.
- Turn off heat.
- Mix well and serve.

Very Berry Smoothie

Ingredients:
- ½ cup raspberries, frozen
- ½ cup blueberries, frozen
- ½ cup strawberries, frozen
- 1 banana
- 1 tbsp. goji berries
  1 tbsp. hemp seed
- 1 cup coconut milk
- Optional: 1 scoop vanilla or chocolate plant-based protein powder.

Instructions:
- Place all ingredients into a high-speed blender.
- Blend until smooth.

222

Chapter 11:
How To Make Everything Meatless

When you first start changing your eating habits you may feel deprived of your favourite comfort foods. The good news is you can still eat them. All you need to do is use plant-based ingredients instead of animal-based ingredients.

Some simple cooking and baking modifications include:

- Replace animal-based saturated fats, like butter, with coconut oil.
- Substitute imitation meat, tofu, beans, lentils or mushrooms in place of meat.
- Use plant-based cheese rather than high-fat dairy cheese.
- Use mustard, or plant-based mayo like Follow Your Heart™ vegenaise, instead of mayonnaise.
- Use fresh herbs to add flavour such as cinnamon, chili powder, basil, oregano and curry.

This vs. That: Ingredient Swap Chart

Ingredient	Vegan Substitution
butter	coconut oil, vegan butter (such as Earth Balance™)
eggs	ground flax or ground chia mixed with water, egg replacer, mashed bananas, apple sauce
meat	tofu, tempeh, seitan, quinoa, lentils, beans, plant-based meats
gelatin	agar, corn starch, arrowroot powder, xanthan gum
honey	maple syrup, agave nectar, coconut sugar
cheese	vegan (nut or soy) cheese, nutritional yeast flakes
mayonnaise	Follow Your Heart™ vegenaise spread, mustard, nut based spread
cow's milk	nut, hemp, rice, soy, coconut milk
ice cream	coconut or soy ice cream, sherbet
yogurt	soy, rice or coconut yogurt

Sample Recipe Modification

In these next two examples you'll see how easy modifying any recipe can be. Choose one of your favourite dishes and make it vegan by using the suggested recipe modifications.

In the recipes, I have not only made the plant-based modifications but also replaced the "not so healthy" ingredients with healthier options.

The good news is, once you know plant-based ingredient options you can take any recipe and transform it into a healthier, plant-based option.

From now on when you see a recipe you like, but it is not plant-based or as healthy as you would like, remember the basic rules above and you'll be able to transform any recipe into a delicious, plant-based meal.

Recipe Modification:
Example #1- Plant-based cheesecake

In this example, you'll see how easy it is to make a plant-based cheesecake. By using healthier ingredients you can make this decadent dessert without all the saturated fat, refined sugar or gluten.

Cheesecake Modification	
Traditional Ingredients	**Plant-Based Ingredients**
Crust:	
•1 ¼ cups graham cracker crumbs •¼ cup margarine •¼ cup sugar	•1 cup raw almonds •1 cup pitted dates •¼ tsp. sea salt
Filling:	
•1 (8 oz.) package cream cheese •1 cup powdered sugar •1 tsp. vanilla extract •1 cup heavy cream, whipped •1 can cherry pie filling	•3 cups cashews, soaked overnight •⅔ cup maple syrup •2 tsp. vanilla powder •⅔ cup raw coconut oil, melted •3 large lemons, peeled •1 cup cherries, pitted
Directions:	
• Mix graham crumbs, margarine and sugar in a bowl until mixed well but still crumbly. • Press into a pie plate. Push crumbs up to the sides of the plate and push into the bottom. •Beat together the cream cheese, sugar and vanilla in a bowl until smooth and spreadable.	• Place almonds, dates and salt in a food processor. Mix until moist. • Press into a pie plate or spring-form pan. Push crumbs up to the sides of the plate and push into the bottom. • Refrigerate until filling is ready.
• Whisk whipped cream into the cream cheese mixture until smooth. • Pour cream cheese into prepared crust. • Smooth the top with a spatula and refrigerate until firm. • Spread the cherry pie filling over the top and refrigerate until ready to serve.	• Rinse cashews and place cashews, maple syrup, vanilla powder, coconut oil, and lemons in a food processor until smooth. • Pour into pan on top of crust. • Chill until set. • Top with fresh cherries.

Recipe Modification:
Example #2 - Lasagna

In this example, you will see how easy it is to make a delicious vegan lasagna by simply replacing the animal-based ingredients with plant-based options.

Lasagna	
Traditional Ingredients	**Plant-Based Modified Ingredients**
• 9-12 lasagna noodles •2 tbsp. olive oil •1 pound lean ground beef •½ onion, diced •½ large bell pepper, diced •2 cloves garlic, minced •1 cup mushrooms, chopped •2 cups spinach, chopped •2, 400 mL cans tomato sauce •⅔ cup tomato paste •1, 400 mL can crushed tomatoes •2 tsp. dried oregano •1 tsp. dried basil •½ tsp. garlic powder •½ tsp. salt •½ tsp. ground black pepper •1 cup ricotta cheese • 2 cups mozzarella cheese, grated	•9-12 lasagna noodles •2 tbsp. coconut oil •1 pound Gardein™ beefless ground •½ onion, chopped •½ large bell pepper, diced •2 cloves garlic, minced •1 cup mushrooms, chopped •2 cups spinach, chopped •2, 400 mL cans tomato sauce •⅔ cup tomato paste •1, 400 mL can crushed tomatoes •2 tsp. dried oregano •1 tsp. dried basil •½ tsp. garlic powder •½ tsp. salt •½ tsp. ground black pepper •1 cup Daiya™ cheddar cheese, grated •2 cups Daiya™ mozzarella cheese, grated
Directions:	
• Preheat oven to 350°F, bring a large pot of water boil cook noodles for 8 to 10 minutes and drain.	• Preheat oven to 350°F, bring a large pot of water boil cook noodles for 8 to 10 minutes and drain.

• Add olive oil to skillet. Heat to medium heat, add beef and cook fully. Drain beef fat. •In another skillet, cook onions, bell pepper, garlic, mushrooms, and spinach with 1 tablespoon olive oil until tender. • Add all remaining ingredients except cheese. Cook until heated. • Combine ricotta and Romano cheese together. • Place layer of sauce at the bottom of a 9×13 inch baking dish. •Top with a layer of noodles, a layer of vegetable mixture and one cup of mozzarella. •Repeat layering until sauce and vegetables mixtures are gone. •Cover with aluminum foil and bake for 60 minutes. • Allow to cool for 15 minutes before serving.	• Add coconut oil to skillet. Heat to medium heat, add beefless ground and cook fully. •In another skillet, cook onions, bell pepper, garlic, mushrooms, and spinach with 1 tablespoon olive oil until tender. • Add all remaining ingredients except cheese. Cook until heated. • Combine vegan cheddar and mozzarella cheese together. • Place layer of sauce at the bottom of a 9×13 inch baking dish. •Top with a layer of noodles, a layer of vegetable mixture and one cup of vegan mozzarella. •Repeat layering until sauce and vegetables mixtures are gone. •Cover with aluminum foil and bake for 60 minutes. • Allow to cool for 15 minutes before serving.

Chapter 12:
Healthy Eating Made Easy

If you are like most people your life is full of personal commitments, including taking care of yourself and making time for your family, friends and professional obligations. This doesn't leave a lot of time to plan and prepare for your meals.

Here are some simple ways to make eating healthy on the run easier:

1) When eating out watch your portion sizes.

It is easy to overeat when in a restaurant. One trick is to order a side dish, rather than a full meal, or put half your meal aside before you start eating to take home to eat another time.

2) Buy lunch at the grocery store.

If you don't have time to make lunch, rather than pulling through the drive through, go to your local grocery store to buy a healthy lunch. You may choose a salad, sandwich, some veggies and

229

hummus or a few pieces of fruit. This will keep you on track with your healthy eating plan and save you money.

3) Cut up and portion out fruits and veggies.

When you've gone to all the trouble of grocery shopping, and purchasing a variety of healthy options, take the time to prepare them when you get home. You will be more likely to eat the fruits and veggies if you wash, peel, chop and store in containers where you can access them more easily than if you just put them in the fridge whole.

This will save you time when you are running out the door and need something to grab and go.

4) Pack a cooler.

When you know you'll be gone most of the day, take some time before you leave the house to pack a cooler with healthy snacks and carry it with you.

It's easy to throw a few things in a bag when you already have them prepared. That way you won't be hungry and tempted to opt for an unhealthy option.

5) Keep healthy snacks handy.

Stock up your car, gym bag or purse, with some non-perishable snacks such as meal replacement shakes, whole food bars, nuts and seeds.

That way if you are running late you have a healthy snack handy to tide you over until you get home. This will curb the temptation to stop for a fast food option.

Eating for long-term health & results:

If you have been accustomed to dieting you may be out of sync with your body and its signals of hunger and fullness.

To get back in balance and to see better results follow these simple guidelines:

1) Eat regularly.

It is important to eat every three-to-four hours. Eat breakfast, lunch and dinner and snacks between these main meals to reduce your hunger. If you ignore your hunger signals this may lead to binge eating later in the day. Eating at regular intervals will reset your clock to a regular pattern of eating and prevent uncontrolled eating.

2) Balance your meals.

Choose a healthy balance of carbohydrates, protein and fat. The American Council of Exercise (ACE) (2014) recommended guidelines suggests that 45 to 65 percent of your diet must come from whole complex carbohydrates. This will provide the body with the energy it needs to function properly and will reduce cravings for sweets.

231

According to ACE, to adequately recover from activity and to repair your body tissues, your balanced diet should consist of 25 to 35 percent protein.

Finally, ACE suggests that the remaining 20 to 25 percent will come from fat for optimal brain, nerve and hormone function. Keep in mind this is only a guideline and optimal balance is based on personal needs and goals.

3) Choose meals and snacks that keep you satisfied.

Eat what you want provided it's a balanced healthy meal. If you eat based on what you think you "should" eat you won't feel satisfied and you risk giving in to cravings.

It's perfectly okay to indulge once in awhile. If you allow yourself to enjoy what you really want to eat, in moderation, you will feel more satisfied and end up eating fewer calories.

4) Listen to your body.

Tune in to your internal cues to hunger rather than external cues such as seeing or smelling food. Learn to eat until you are satisfied rather than after you are stuffed. The easiest way to get in the habit of doing this is to take smaller portions and eat slowly and mindfully.

5) Enjoy your food.

When eating, take the time to pay full attention to the food. Stay present and allow yourself to taste, notice the texture and savour the food without guilt. Have fun. Experiment with your food. Try new recipes to prevent boredom.

A BEGINNERS GUIDE TO GOING MEATLESS

Chapter 13:
Living The Meatless Lifestyle

Up until this point, most of the information I have shared with you has been about food. However, there is more to living a conscious and compassionate life than just eating plant-based food.

Embracing a vegan lifestyle means not using any products tested on or use animals in any way, getting involved in the community and being a role model to inspire others to do the same.

Use Vegan Products

Getting rid of everything in your home that is not vegan may take a little more time to embrace, especially since many products you use on a daily basis are in some way made from animal products.

Like the transition to plant-based food, moving away from all animal products can happen one-step-at-a-time.

235

Take some time to educate yourself about what products contain animals and seek products that have a vegan, or cruelty-free, label.

Some products that are made with animals include:

- Make-up
- Shampoo, conditioner and body-care products
- Nail polish
- Cologne and perfume
- Toothpaste
- Candles
- Condoms
- Crayons
- Fabric softener
- Cars
- Clothing
- Shoes

According to PETA some ingredients found in these products, and more, that have been derived from animals include:

- **Albumen** is found in cosmetics, derived from egg whites and used as a coagulating agent.

- **Alpha-Hydroxy Acid**, or lactic acid, is most often derived from animals and is often used in anti-aging products.

- **Ambergris** is made from whale intestines and is used in perfumes and food and beverages.

- **Biotin** comes from milk and yeast and is used in cosmetics, shampoos and creams.

- **Carmine, Cochineal, Carminic Acid** is the red pigment from crushed cochineal insect and is used in cosmetics, shampoo and in foods for colouring.

- **Down** is another word for goose or duck feathers and is used in clothing and bedding.

- **Fur,** taken from a variety of animals, is used for clothing and decor.

- **Gelatin** is made from the skin, tendons, ligaments and bones of animals and used as a binder in shampoo, cosmetics and food products.

- **Glycerin or glycerol** is from animal fat, unless specified as vegetable glycerin, and is used in cosmetics, gum, medicines, soaps and lubricants.

- **Guanine**, from fish scales, is used in cosmetics, nail polish and shampoo.

- **Insulin**, excreted from hog pancreas, is used as medicine for diabetics.

- **Isinglass** is another name for fish bladders and is often used to filter alcoholic beverages like wine and beer.

- **Keratin** is made from ground up horns, hooves and feathers and is used in shampoos and other hair products.

- **Lanolin** is made from the oil glands of sheep and used in skin-care products, cosmetics and medicines.

- **Leather** is usually made from cow, or other, animal skin and used for clothing, vehicles and furniture.

- **Musk (oil)** is the secretion obtained from musk deer, beaver and other animals and used in perfumes and food flavourings.

- **Pepsin** is found in hogs' stomachs and used as a clotting agent in some cheese and vitamins.

- **Rennet** is an enzyme from calves' stomachs used in cheese making.

- **Shellac** is the excretion of certain insects and is used in candy, hair and nail lacquer and jewelry.

- **Squalene** is the oil from shark livers and is used in cosmetics, moisturizers and hair dyes.

- **Stearyl Alcohol** can be prepared from sperm whales and is found in medicine, hair and body-care products.

I agree, looking at this list can be overwhelming. Cutting out all of this may seem like an impossible task. Just pay attention to where your products come from and do your best to stay away from anything animal-based.

For example, look at your clothing and get rid of, or choose to no longer purchase, coats made with fur trim or down feathers, wallets or purses made of leather, or boots made of leather or fur trim.

If you already have these items you may choose to give them away or keep them and bless the animal that gave its life for the item, respect the item and choose to replace it, when it's time, with a vegan option.

It is easy today to choose clothing items that are vegan since many new vegan specific companies are now in business and choose more compassionate business practices.

It's not about being perfect. I know I'm not! What's more important is that you now make more conscious choices to minimize the cruel practices animals endure to make these products.

Get Involved

A great way to truly embrace the vegan lifestyle is to get involved in the community.

Look in your area and seek out vegan potlucks, community meet-ups or animal activism events. You might even choose to find an animal sanctuary or rescue organization that could use your help.

Attending these types of events, and volunteering with rescue organizations, allows you to connect with others who have made the same lifestyle choice and will be a great support system for you.

Be A Role Model

Just by making the choice to embrace a vegan lifestyle you are already a role model to others. By simply living your life in this way people will begin to notice a shift in you.

You don't need to educate or preach to others about going vegan to make a difference. Just live your life and be the change you want to see in the world. Actions speak much louder than words.

Vote With Your Dollars

How you choose to spend your money represents your core values. Your core values are those important to you such as your family, health and animal welfare.

When you spend your money to purchase a product or service, the company sees this as a vote. You are saying YES to wanting more of that product or service and they will continue to produce more of what you want. Therefore, it's important to think about who and what you're supporting when you make a purchase of any kind.

I remember when I was just starting my journey to a vegan lifestyle all I really thought about was the food I was eating and not much else. This was hard enough. However, after learning more about what companies are doing to get their products to market I started to question whether or not I agreed with what they were doing. In other words, did their core values align with mine?

In the next section, you will learn how to vote with your dollars without compromising your values.

1) Clarify Your Core Values

Core values are the rules you choose to live by. They're the non-negotiable things you have decided are important to you. For example, you may value health, your freedom, money, your family, animals and human rights and there's nothing that could get you to compromise on these values.

Activity:

1) Take a moment to write down the top 10 things you think are the most important to you in your life right now.

2) When you complete this list circle the top five most important values from your top 10.

3) Write down these top values in order of importance.

For example, my top 10 values are:

1. Health
2. Freedom
3. Money
4. Family
5. Animal welfare
6. Integrity
7. Connection
8. Adventure
9. Compassion
10. Respect

My top five values, in order of importance, are:

1. Health
2. Freedom
3. Money
4. Family
5. Compassion

Remember, your core values may change over time so it's important to revisit and revise them often.

2) Identify The Companies You Buy From

Most people who live in North America buy products and services on a regular basis but barely give any thought to who these companies are or what their core values are.

If you choose to live a compassionate, plant-based lifestyle and don't want to contribute to animal cruelty or the destruction of our beautiful planet, wouldn't it be wise to make sure the products and services you buy do not go to companies that do support these things?

For example, let's take a look at make-up companies. The cosmetic industry is a multi-billion dollar industry; however, before many products hit the public market they go through extensive testing on animals to be sure they are safe for human use. Sadly, these tests are often very painful and cause much suffering to the animals.

Therefore, if you wear make-up and your values include compassion and animal welfare, it's important to be sure these companies are not testing on animals.

Check out PETA's blog for a list of cosmetic companies that test on animals: https://www.peta.org/living/personal-care-fashion/beauty-brands-that-you-thought-were-cruelty-free-but-arent/.

Activity:

1) Go through your house and write down a list of all the major brands you use and companies you support. This includes food, cleaning products, make-up and clothing.

2) Make a list of all the services you use such as

getting your hair and nails done, coaching and any other service-based businesses.

3) Do an Internet search to see what best practices these companies use to develop their products.

When I made my own list years ago I began to look deeper into the companies I was buying from. After doing my research and learning more about these companies I chose to let some of the products go and support other, more vegan-friendly and healthier brands.

3) Decide If The Company's Values And Your Values Align

Once you have the list of your own core values and the companies you support, take a look to see if your values align with theirs.

I realized, after doing my own personal search that some of the companies I was supporting, did not do things in a way that aligned with my own core values. That is when I decided to research products and services from companies whose values align better with my own.

I was astonished to find out that many of the companies I was supporting used a variety of chemical ingredients known to be carcinogenic, such as sodium laurel sulphate in toothpaste and aluminum in deodorant. At the time, I had no idea these ingredients were that bad for my health until I

244

started to do more research.

Other companies were doing animal testing or were cruel to animals in the production of their products. I knew at that moment I had to change my ways.

Activity:

Ask yourself a series of questions based on your own core values to discover if each company is one you want to keep supporting or if it's time to find another one to support.

Questions may include:

1. Does this company believe in ethical sourcing of ingredients or do they contribute to animal cruelty and destruction of the environment?

2. Does this company support human slavery such as poor working conditions and below fair pay for employees?

3. Does this company test their products on animals or humans that cause suffering, disease and death?

4. Does this company contribute to the community in a positive way or do they take away from the community?

The answers to these questions, and how you choose to proceed, are ultimately based what you believe to be acceptable corporate practices.

4) Choose To Buy Products From Companies Whose Values Align With Your Own

After doing this research, you now have a choice to make. You can either turn your head to unethical behaviours and poor practices from these companies or you can refuse to support them.

If the company in question has core values or business practices that align with your own and you feel that supporting them will make the world a better place, that's great! Keep supporting these companies and recommend them to as many people as you can. This will help them grow and keep doing good things in the world.

If the company has core values or business practices that do not align with yours, then you know what to do. Stop supporting these companies immediately because the more money you give to them the bigger they get and the more they think it's okay to keep doing what they're doing.

For example, if you are buying meat products from a company that is cruel to their animals and causes them to suffer while they're alive, and during their death, then you are saying, "YES," I support this behaviour.

However, if you choose to no longer purchase animal products, you are saying, "NO," to these practices and the companies that provide these products will eventually be forced to stop selling them.

Activity:

From now on, before you purchase any product or service, research the company and its best practices as much as you can to be sure you are supporting a company that isn't harming you, another living being or the environment.

By being a more conscious, informed consumer you are contributing to the protection of all living things and upgrading the world in which we live.

Always remember, with every choice you make, every purchase, every action, you're voting with your dollars. You are either saying, "YES," I support you or, "NO," I do not support you!

Now the question is, "who and what will you support?"

A BEGINNERS GUIDE TO GOING MEATLESS

Getting Started

By feeding your body with plant-based food you are giving yourself permission to treat your body with the love and respect it deserves.

By choosing to no longer use products and services that contribute to the suffering of animals, or destruction of the planet, you are being a responsible citizen of the world who cares about making this world a better place for future generations.

Over time, you will watch your body, mind, soul and life transform before your eyes.

Remember, this lifestyle choice is not about being perfect. It's about taking simple steps when you are ready and being kind to yourself even if things aren't as perfect as you would like them to be.

You may choose to become vegan overnight or take it slowly. Either way, congratulations on having the courage to do something not many people are able to do. Going against the grain is how all change happens.

Remember, you have chosen this lifestyle out of compassion for yourself and for animals. However, other humans, regardless of their personal beliefs, actions or choices still deserve your compassion and love. At times this might be hard but it is necessary to cultivate more compassion and love, which is necessary for this world to become a better place.

Please visit **www.livingmeatless.com** to stay updated on the latest vegan health and nutrition information, courses and book releases.

I wish you much love and blessings,

Rachel Joy Olsen, BSc. MBA
Plant-Based Nutrition, Health & Wellness Coach
www.livingmeatless.com

Resources

To succeed on this incredible journey, take time to continually educate yourself about the vegan lifestyle and why it is recommend by top health and wellness professionals in the world.

Below are some resources that I referenced to write this book or I recommend to check out for further information on this topic.

Documentaries:

My favourite documentaries that review the health benefits of a plant-based lifestyle include:

- **The Game Changers:** This is the newest documentary, released in 2019, that highlights the benefits of plant-based diet for athletic performance. https://gamechangersmovie.com

- **Forks Over Knives:** This documentary presents the plant-based diet as a cure for many of the most common chronic diseases. https://www.forksoverknives.com

251

- **Vegucated.** This documentary follows six people testing out a vegan diet for six weeks. https://www.getvegucated.com

- **Eating You Alive.** This documentary focuses on curing chronic disease with a plant-based diet. https://www.eatingyoualive.com

- **Food Choices.** Documents the effects our food choices have on our health, the animals, and the planet. http://www.foodchoicesmovie.com

- **What The Health.** This documentary focuses on the debilitating chronic diseases and how a plant-based diet has the potential to completely change the health of a nation and the world. https://www.whatthehealthfilm.com

- **Plant Pure Nation.** This documentary highlights the importance of a whole-food, plant-based diet for health along with the challenges in bringing that message to mainstream society. https://www.plantpurenation.com

- **Chow Down.** The journey of three people who attempt to reverse their heart disease and diabetes by adhering to a plant-based diet. https://www.fmtv.com/watch/chow-down

- **Hungry For Change.** Uncovers the secrets to vibrant health and lasting weight loss. http://www.hungryforchange.tv

Documentaries featuring animals and their cruel treatment include:

- **Earthlings:** An American documentary film about humankind's total dependence on animals for economic purposes. *http://www.nationearth.com*

- **Blackfish:** A documentary that features the captivity of Tilikum, an orca involved in the deaths of three individuals, and the consequences of keeping orcas in captivity. *https://www.netflix.com/ca/title/70267802*

- **The Cove:** A documentary that analyzes, and questions the dolphin hunting practices in Japan. *https://www.opsociety.org/our-work/films/the-cove/*

- **I Am An Animal: The Story of Ingrid Newkirk:** A documentary about the beliefs and motives of the British co-founder and driving force behind the Ethical Treatment of Animals (PETA), the worlds' largest animal rights organization. *https://www.peta2.com/news/i-am-an-animal/*

- **Food Inc.:** A film that examines America's unflattering corporate controlled food industry. *https://www.netflix.com/ca/title/70108783*

- **Speciesism:** A documentary that takes views on a frightening look into the hidden side of factory farming.
  https://speciesismthemovie.com

Documentaries that highlight how our current choices effect the environment include:

- **Cowspiracy:** This documentary uncovers the most destructive industry facing the planet today – and investigates why the world's leading environmental organizations are too afraid to talk about it.
  http://www.cowspiracy.com

- **Racing Extinction:** This documentary exposes the issues of endangered species and mass extinction. *https://racingextinction.com*

- **Virunga:** The true story of a group of brave individuals who risk their lives to save Africa's oldest national park. *https://virungamovie.com*

- **Last Days of Ivory:** This is an animated short documentary film about the decline of African elephant populations and the illegal ivory trade.
  http://www.lastdaysofivory.com

- **Chasing Ice:** This documentary is the story of one man's mission to change the tide of history by gathering undeniable evidence of our changing planet. *https://chasingice.com*

Books:

This list of books will help enhance your knowledge on the subject of becoming vegan:

- *21-Day Weight Loss Kickstart* – Dr. Neil Barnard w

- *30-Day Vegan Challenge* - Colleen Patrick-Goudreau

- *The China Study* - Dr. T. Colin Campbell

- *Conscious Eating* - Dr. Gabriel Cousins

- *Eat More, Weigh Less* - Dean Ornish, MD

- *Eating Animals* - Jonathan Safran Foer

- *Forks Over Knives* - Gene Stone

- **How Not To Die** - Dr. Michael Greger with Gene Stone

- *Living Foods For Optimal Health* - Dr. Brian Clement

- *Prevent and Reverse Heart Disease* - Dr. Caldwell B. Esselstyn, Jr. MD

- *Quantum Wellness* - Kathy Freston

255

- *Skinny Bitch* - Rory Freedman and Kim Bornouin

- *The Food Revolution* - John Robbins

- *The Kind Diet* - Alicia Silverstone

- *Thrive* - Brendan Brazier

- *Vegan: The New Ethics of Eating* - Erik Marcus

Websites:

- Hippocrates Health Institute: **http://hippocratesinst.org/**

- Living Meatless Nutrition & Wellness: **https://livingmeatless.com**

- Nutrition Facts: **http://nutritionfacts.org/**

- Physicians Committee For Responsible Medicine: **https://www.pcrm.org**

- The Real Truth About Health: **http://www.therealtruthabouthealth.com/**

References

1. **American Cancer Society (2015).** World Health Organization Says Processed Meat Causes Cancer. https://www.cancer.org/latest-news/world-health-organization-says-processed-meat-causes-cancer.html

2. **American Council On Exercise (2013).** ACE Health Coach Manual: The Ultimate Guide To Wellness, Fitness & Lifestyle Change.

3. **American Council On Exercise (2014).** American Council On Exercise Personal Trainer Manual (5 ed.).

4. **American Heart Association (2015).** Dietary Fat Recommendations 1957-2015: Focus Shifts Form Total Fat To Type Of Fat. https://www.heart.org/-/media/files/healthy-living/company-collaboration/inap/dietary-fat-recommendations-timeline-pdf-ucm_474998.pdf

5. **American Heart Association (2015).** Saturated Fat: AHA Recommendation. https://www.heart.org/en/healthy-living/healthy-eating/eat-smart/fats/saturated-fats

6. **Axe, J. Dr. (2018).** Top 10 High Antioxidant Foods. https://draxe.com/nutrition/article/top-10-high-antioxidant-foods/

7. **Campbell, Dr. T. Colin & Campbell II, Dr. Thomas M. (2006).** The China Study: Startling Implications For Diet, Weight Loss and Long-Term Health.

8. **Clement, B., PhD. (2014).** Killer Fish: How Eating Aquatic Life endangers Your Health.

9. **Clement, B., PhD. (1998).** Living Foods For Optimum Health: Your Complete Guide To The Healing Power Of Raw Foods.

10. **Cousins, G., Dr. (2005).** Spiritual Nutrition. https://www.drcousensonlinestore.com/Dr-Cousens-Spiritual-Nutrition-p/437.htm

11. **Craig, W., Mangels, A.R., & American Dietetic Association (2009).** Position of The American Dietetic Association: Vegetarian Diets. PubMed.gov. https://www.ncbi.nlm.nih.gov/pubmed/19562864

12. **D'Adamo, P., Dr. (1996).** Eat Right For Your Type. https://dadamo.com/txt/index.pl?0000

13. **Diabetes Canada (2013).** Glycemic Index Food Guide. https://guidelines.diabetes.ca/docs/patient-resources/glycemic-index-food-guide.pdf

14. **Esselstyne. C., Dr. (2007).** Prevent and Reverse Heart Disease. http://www.dresselstyn.com

15. **Freston, K. (2011).** The Breathtaking Effects Of Cutting Back On Meat. https://www.huffpost.com/entry/the-breathtaking-effects_b_181716

16. **Government Of Canada (2019).** Canada's Food Guide. https://food-guide.canada.ca/en/

17. **Greger, M., Dr. (2014).** Eat Beans To Live Longer. https://nutritionfacts.org/2014/09/16/eat-beans-to-live-longer/

18. **Greger, M., Dr. (2019).** How Not To Die. https://nutritionfacts.org/book/

19. **Greger, M. Dr. (2018).** The Risk Of Fish Oil Supplements. https://nutritionfacts.org/2018/02/20/the-risks-of-fish-oil-supplements/

20. **Greger, M., Dr. (2017).** Why Is Milk Consumption Associated With More Bone Fractures? https://nutritionfacts.org/2017/01/31/why-is-milk-consumption-associated-with-more-bone-fractures/

21. **Haytowitz, D. & Bhagwat, S. (2010).** USDA Database For The Oxygen Radical Absorbency Capacity (ORAC) Of Selected Foods. http://www.orac-info-portal.de/download/ORAC_R2.pdf

22. **The Humane Society of The United States (2019).** An HSUS Fact Sheet: Greenhouse Gas

Emissions From Animal Agriculture. https://
www.humanesociety.org/sites/default/files/
archive/assets/pdfs/farm/hsus-fact-sheet-
greenhouse-gas-emissions-from-animal-
agriculture.pdf

23. **Imatome-Yun, N. (2016).** Why The Standard
American Diet Is Even Sadder Then We Thought.
https://www.forksoverknives.com/standard-
american-diet-sadder-than-we-thought/#gs.lfpyc9

24. **Kawakhito, S. Kitahata, H. Oshita, S. (2009).**
Problems Associated With Glucose Toxicity: Role
Of Hyperglycemia-Induced Oxidative Stress.
https://www.ncbi.nlm.nih.gov/pmc/articles/
PMC2738809/

25. **Mercola, J., Dr. (2016).** What Are The Health
Benefits Of Coconut Oil?
https://articles.mercola.com/health-benefits-
coconut-oil.aspx

26. **The National Academies of Sciences
Engineering Medicine (2002).** Dietary Reference
Intakes for Energy, Carbohydrate, Fiber, Fat, Fatty
Acids, Cholesterol, Protein, and Amino Acids.
http://www.nationalacademies.org/hmd/Reports/
2002/Dietary-Reference-Intakes-for-Energy-
Carbohydrate-Fiber-Fat-Fatty-Acids-Cholesterol-
Protein-and-Amino-Acids.aspx

27. **National Cancer Institute (2017).** Chemicals In
Meat Cooked At High Temperatures and Cancer

Risk. https://www.cancer.gov/about-cancer/
causes-prevention/risk/diet/cooked-meats-fact-
sheet

28. **Obesity Canada (2019).** Obesity In Canada.
https://obesitycanada.ca/obesity-in-canada/

29. **Patrick-Goudreau, C. (2016).** Food For Thought
Podcast: If The World Went Vegan, We Would Be
Overrun With Animals and Other Hypotheticals.
https://www.colleenpatrickgoudreau.com/if-the-
world-went-vegan-we-would-be-overrun-with-
animals-and-other-hypotheticals/

30. **PETA (2019).** Meat and the Environment. https://
www.peta.org/issues/animals-used-for-food/meat-
environment/

31. **PETA (2019).** Starter Kit: Everything You Need To
Eat Right For Your Health, For Animals, And For
The Earth. https://www.peta.org/living/food/free-
vegan-starter-kit/

32. **Physicians Committee For Responsible
Medicine.** https://www.pcrm.org.

33. **Potgieter, S. (2012).** Sport Nutrition: A Review Of
The Latest Guidelines For Exercise And Sport
Nutrition From The American College Of Sport
Nutrition, The International Olympic Committee
And The International Society For Sport Nutrition.
https://www.overvoedingengezondheid.nl/wp-
content/uploads/2015/03/88379-219821-1-PB.pdf

34. **Robertson, R., PhD. (2017).** Omega 3-6-9 Fatty Acids: A Complete Overview. https://www.healthline.com/nutrition/omega-3-6-9-overview

35. **Sanders, B. (2018).** Global Animal Statistics and Charts. https://faunalytics.org/global-animal-slaughter-statistics-and-charts/

36. **Scarborough, P., Appleby, P.N., Mizdrak, A. et al. Climatic Change (2014)** 125:179. Dietary Greenhouse Gas Emissions Of Meat-Eaters, Fish-Eaters, Vegetarians and Vegans In The UK. https://doi.org/10.1007/s10584-014-1169-1

37. **Science (2018).** Meat Consumption, Health And The Environment. https://science.sciencemag.org/content/361/6399/eaam5324

38. **Science Daily (2018).** E. Coli Strain From Retail Poultry May Cause Urinary Tract Infections In People. https://www.sciencedaily.com/releases/2018/08/180828085911.htm

39. **Schwalfenberg, G.K. (2012).** The Alkaline Diet: Is There Evidence That An Alkaline pH Diet Benefits Health? J. Environ Public Health. 2012;2012:727630. Doi:10. 1155/2012/727630. https://www.ncbi.nlm.nih.gov/pmc/articles/PMC3195546/

40. **Statistics Canada (2015).** Overweight and Obese Adults (self-Reported), 2014.

https://www150.statcan.gc.ca/n1/pub/82-625-x/
2015001/article/14185-eng.htm

41. **University of Arizona (2003).** The Chemistry of
Amino Acids. http://www.biology.arizona.edu/
biochemistry/problem_sets/aa/aa.html

42. **Vancouver Humane Society (2015).** Almost 12
Million Canadians Now Vegetarian or Trying To
Eat Less Meat.
http://www.vancouverhumanesociety.bc.ca/
almost-12-million-canadians-now-vegetarian-or-
trying-to-eat-less-meat/

43. **The Vegan Society (2019).** The Honey Industry.
https://www.vegansociety.com/go-vegan/honey-
industry

About The Author

Rachel Joy Olsen, BSc., MBA believes that whole- food nutrition and living a compassionate lifestyle are the secrets to healthy bliss. Her passion is to inspire people to embrace ultimate health and wellness as their number one priority and achieve the life they desire.

She is the author of a variety of nutrition and wellness books and founder of R.J.O. Wellness & Academy and Living Meatless Nutrition & Wellness.

Rachel is a health and wellness coach, weight management and exercise specialist, yoga instructor, certified raw vegan nutritionist and chef, who has been inspiring people for over two decades.

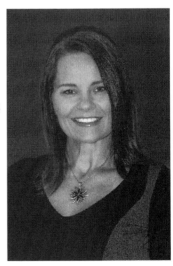

She offers online and in-person courses, coaching programs and workshops to assist her clients on their journey to an upgraded life.

Photo by K.J. Pictures, 4-13 Studios

Made in the USA
Columbia, SC
06 December 2019